Praise for The Poetry

"Perfect for solitary contemplation, this anthology is full of yogic wisdom."

–Yoga Journal Magazine

"This book is a link that paints an important picture and gives us that experience of looking beyond appearances and feeling that profound parallel between the yogic experience and poetry."

–Rod Stryker

"This book is the soul ignited."

–Sianna Sherman

"These beautiful poems speak to and are expressions of the very heart of yoga."

–Kelly Birch, Editor, Yoga Therapy Today

"To have yoga without poetry is like having marriage without love. Poetry is the essence of beauty in language. I am grateful for HawaH having put together this volume to inspire yoga students with the beauty of meter and verse."

–Aadil Palkhivala, Master Yoga Teacher

"This collection of poems is a beautiful expression of the collective consciousness of the modern day yoga culture."

–YOGANONYMOUS

"As I started to scan through the pages, I felt like I had won the lottery! Like a beautiful asana, each page contains words perfectly aligned to lift my soul. I had been given the gift of a book of yoga poems that I know will provide inspiration for my life and my yoga classes for many years to come."

–The Daily Downward Dog

"This book is a sweet gift offering to any poetically inclined yoga practitioner and a perfect item to have at yoga studios. Often, instructors will be able to bring resting students back from Savasana with an inspiring reading. *The Poetry of Yoga* offers a trove of fresh selections. Like asana practice itself, each visit to the book will bring new discovery and communion."

–Mount Shasta Magazine

"It is such an incredible combination of yoga and poetry that we were literally 'blown away.' It has so many great poems and the offerings from the yoga community makes us proud and happy to be a part of something so special."

–Flow Yoga Magazine

"This book is successfully building momentum to revitalize the ancient tradition of yoga poetry."

–Art of Zen Yoga

"*The Poetry of Yoga* is an amazing book. . .featuring some of today's greatest yoga teachers!"

–Opposing Views

"*The Poetry of Yoga* anthology harnesses the energy of a great movement of healing arts practitioners. . .and crossed the lines to gather and contribute 21st century reflections of the state of an ancient practice. . ."

–Tribe

"I used to dream about living in the desert, where the mountains turned pink at sunset, snow graced mountain tops, and every star and galaxy in the sky opened its glimmering eyes; now it is all here in an anthology!"

–Sister Hawk

"A powerhouse book of poems!"

–Where is My Guru

"Heartwarming, funny, inspiring and enlightening. A great collection for poetry lovers—whether you practice yoga or not!"

–Chelsea Edgett

"Lots of people write and read poetry and we should all come out of the closet about it."

–Mind Body Green

"A monumental work of art, compiled and offered as a global reflection. The many poems, colors, perceptions and cadences, in *The Poetry of Yoga* together stand as one glowing source of light. . .one representing our generation."

–Hosh Yoga

"When you're a child and read Dr. Seuss, poetry becomes part of the childhood landscape. This is a playful, contemplative, whimsical, serious gateway back to that place. Rhyme or not, long or short, this collection of poems skewers the heart and spirit with a joyful edge. It's a must-have for any library!"

–Sherry Hanck

"I'm impressed, there is actually a whole, budding theory on how yoga and creativity can work together in all kinds of mediums, from writing, to painting, to music, or just dealing with issues coming up in whatever work it is you do. We need creativity in all aspects of our lives, and in order to access it, we have to be willing to step out of our comfortable boxes."

–Spirituality and Health

"This book is a great victory. A voice to contemporary yoga. Through this book we get to see the somatic power of consciousness."

–Shiva Rea

the poetry of YOGA

Light Pouring from Pens

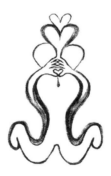

Edited By HawaH

Invocation By Shiva Rea

WHITE CLOUD PRESS
ASHLAND, OREGON

White Cloud Press books may be purchased for educational, business, or sales promotional use. For information, please write:

Special Market Department
White Cloud Press
PO Box 3400
Ashland, OR 97520
Website: www.whitecloudpress.com

Cover and Interior Design by C Book Services

First edition: 2014
14 15 16 17 18   10 9 8 7 6 5 4 3 2 1

Printed in the United States of America

Library of Congress Cataloging-in-Publication Data

The poetry of yoga : light pouring from pens / edited by HawaH ; invocation by Shiva Rea. -- First edition.
    pages cm. -- (Poetry of yoga series ; 1)
  ISBN 978-1-940468-25-9 (paperback)
1. Poetry--21st century. 2. Yoga--Poetry. 3. Spiritual life--Poetry. I. HawaH. II. Rea, Shiva.
PN6101.P5445 2014
808.81--dc23
                                    2014029368

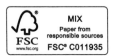

MIX
Paper from
responsible sources
FSC
www.fsc.org   FSC® C011935

Ring the bells that still can ring
Forget your perfect offering
There is a crack in everything
That's how the light gets in.

–Leonard Cohen

Contents

Compassion

Desire

Freedom

Transformation

Service

Invocation

This book
you hold in your hands
comes from breathing bodies.

Tenderized through the fire of yoga
transformed by moments and
years of practice and
letting go into the natural flow.

It can happen to anyone
when you least expect it
the creative fire arrow releases
in the middle of a meditation
a wide open asana
or a deep embrace
while you were turning the corner
or dressing your child
or calling out in kirtan
falling down
rising up
cracking open
exhaling as freedom born again.

The sages say,
You can teach science to anyone and turn them
Into a master.
But not even a Guru can awaken the flow of poetry.
It releases spontaneously from within.

This inner creative fire of yoga
churns life experiences
into poetic shakti
with the power
to ignite the dormant
dissolve barriers
and sustain connection to your deepest source.

This book will hold you
as the poets of each page become
intimate friends,
guiding you through the inner landscape
echoing a wisdom teaching,
a tenderness,
a mirror of your own truth.

If you become receptive inside
you can work with this book like a mala
each poem an offering
arising at the right time like a precious jewel
remembering what was lost, forgotten or hidden.

This book is a great victory
a celebration
for the cells who carried the creative spark through time
for the Sages who poured the nectar of realization
into the hymns, songs and sutras that were the poetry of
the Vedas, Upanishads, Gita, Tantraloka.

These poems are not lost in post-modern translation
but alive with the current of all poets who have vibrated their
truth in treacherous times.

These poems are a tribute to those extraordinary poetic
teachers such as Kabir, Lalla, Mirabai, Rumi, and Tagore
whose teachings wrapped in love songs to the Divine
helped us become more human.

May all who hold this book be transformed
by the twilight language of poetry
that bows to the eternal in a million different ways.

Each poem will find you at the right moment and bring
you closer to the author and also your Self.

In a world that is trying to find a compass
to navigate rough waters ahead,
Poetry is the unexpected divining rod,
a nadi line between time
an ear to the ancestors
a yoga practice for the soul.

To honor the poetic revelation, revolution and evolution
that our brave editor, HawaH calls forth:

May you take up a new or old yoga sadhana with a pen
And blank page.
Bend your outer mind into your heart.
Inhale the fire that waits for us all.
Write a poem from your breathing body
and feel the yoga of poetry. . .

Shiva Rea

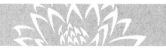

Prologue

I've been practicing yoga and writing poetry since I was a small child. Fascinated by the rhythm of verse, I started writing around the age of eight with my sister in the back seat of our family car. A couple years older than me, she stared intently out the window composing rhymes of passing birds and clouds. Ever since that day, poetry has danced in my blood.

Yoga, similarly, was inspired from a family member; in this case, my mom. A devout Hindu, she encased Hanuman and Ganesh in picture frames above my bed. Back then she taught me different mantras to chant during prayers and ceremonies. I guess you can say I first began my journey to yoga through Bhakti.

When not diving into my yoga practice, I am often found with pencil in hand, scribbling down a poem, or nose in a book, reading ancient poetic verse. The two seem rather inseparable, since many sacred texts were communicated through poetry, including the Bhagavad Gita, The Tao Te Ching, and the Holy Quran. I feel affinity toward the power of poetry in transforming lives, and in a similar way, witnessed my own life changed by yoga.

Doing yoga pushes me inside, and writing helps me communicate outwardly. I was moved by the creative possibilities of knitting together the two and wanted to share this love and passion with others. In 2009, I started developing a workshop called *The Poetry of Yoga*, doing just that. To get the formula right, I taught it a few times in my hometown of Washington, D.C., and then took it on tour by the summer of 2010. In the beginning I had no plans of pulling together a book. I was visiting cities throughout the country, encouraging people to write poetry while doing yoga. Each workshop proved a powerful outpouring beyond my expectations. During the workshop, I would teach sequences of asana broken up with creative writing prompts. At climatic moments participants wrote poetry while actually in asana.

In the first two hours, we completed a dynamic asana sequence, after which the participants wrote a few poems about their feelings and experiences during their practice. The next hour we spent in a circle, sharing all we had written. In many cases, the sharing put most of us in tears and proved instrumental to the process of transformation and healing. In the final thirty minutes, I did a spoken word poetry performance that framed service, love, peace, healing, suffering, sustainability, and freedom. About half way through the tour, I realized the soul-stirring poetry we were creating had to be shared with others. And so, was birthed, *The Poetry of Yoga* book idea.

The new mission I charged myself with was to help kick-start and harness a modern day renaissance of Hafiz, Mirabai, and Rumi. I figured I could do this through expanding the literary tradition of yoga to include the cultural perspective of the 21st century.

Most of the celebrated mystic poet yogis have long been deceased. I envisioned the book as a platform for a new body of work reflecting on how yoga continues to shift the landscape of human consciousness and civilization. A book anthology of modern-living poetic voices was exactly what I was being called to create. I knew they were living amongst us, and simply needed a platform to share their existential expressions.

Here began the effortless unfolding. Sure there was lots of work involved, but in the larger scheme of things this project took on a life of its own. I began to accept online submissions of poetry in October of 2010 for the book. Over the next six months I received over 1,500 pages of poetry from 16 different countries. The outpouring of breath-giving poetry revealed that I was not the only one with this idea. There came a point, during the final week of submissions, when over 35 poems were submitted each day! I officially closed submissions on April 15, 2011.

To supplement and excite people about the idea, I asked living master teachers and writers from around the world to also contribute poetry to the project. I wanted to get their voices in the mix, and began sending out invitation letters over email to those I knew. I planned to integrate and combine the words of established teachers with everyday people, as well as participants who attended *The Poetry of Yoga* workshops.

In order to land such an all-star cast of featured writers, I delicately persisted. . .over and over and over again. It wasn't enough to send emails, so I traveled, went to workshops, and met the practitioners I wanted to include in the anthology. In person, I told them about my idea and asked if they would participate and help.

I was struck by the awesome response from the established teachers. The only time someone said, "No," was in their adamancy that they didn't write poetry. Interestingly enough, one of my goals was to encourage yoga teachers and students to step out of their comfort zones and write poetry, even if they had never done so in the past.

I felt this was a very important piece to the puzzle. I believe extensive schooling in one specific subject area creates a boundary of pre-condition, limiting one's creative and expressive capacity. This often sets unimaginative parameters on how you think something is supposed to sound, taste, touch, or feel. Some of the most brilliant and beautiful poetry I've read is from people who have never written a poem before. It's fresh, new, and contains a perspective devoid of this pre-conditioning. If you have ever read anything by Picasso you know exactly what I mean. He's a painter, but when he wrote. . .his words rang with an eloquence, breathing clarity, conciseness, and creativity that a thoroughbred writer would find hard to achieve.

And so I fished for poetry from the far reaches of the globe. . .searching for the undiscovered modern day Rumis and Hafizs, posting the International Call for Submissions on websites, list-serves, and using social marketing tools to get the word out. It seems it might have worked. A litany of emails started coming through the comments page on the website; personal emails I received from people expressed that the project inspired them to write their first poem ever; others spoke to the timeliness of such an anthology. What began as a one-human guerrilla operation became a poetic movement, harnessing social media for extensive outreach in gathering a plethora of submissions.

The reading of all the poetry that came in has been an absolute pleasure and joy. It was an honor to have my finger on the pulse of such creative, soul-inspiring, and mystical poetry from around the world. It took months to read the work over and over again. I've been doing this while on the train (staring out the window between poems to catch my breath), while sitting in Upavistha Konasana in my meditation room (burning sage and watching the flickering candle light dance across words), while at the park (serenaded by drum circles), while at the coffee shop (smelling the aroma of awakening), and while sitting in the doctor's waiting room (no hurry, I was reading patience).

I've created distance and space by reading the same poems in different environments, seeing how they affected me at different times. Making the decision about what would appear in this collection was a monumental task. In order to protect any bias, I read the poetry without seeing the names of the authors. After reading and sorting the work into large piles through an internal system of poetic theme and quality, I began to move poetry from pile to pile. Slowly I narrowed the work down to 450 pages, still too much for one book! It seemed unfair to try and limit the work to one anthology. So I decided to turn the submitted poetry into two anthologies and make use of this opportunity to broadcast to the world all these tremendous poetic voices.

I included poems from Sri Lanka, Ireland, Philippines, China, Wales, Guatemala, India, Norway, U.S.A., Australia, Japan, Pakistan, Romania, Mexico, England, South Africa, Brazil, Canada, etc. . .to assure the anthology contained a diverse chorus of voices that represented different geographical regions of the world.

My editing preference was to also value and honor diversity of theme. Some of the hardest decisions to make were filtering poems touching on the same theme. For example, it's possible someone wrote a brilliant poem about "breath" that was not accepted because a third of the poems explored the theme of breath. To keep the book balanced I only included a handful of poems on breath, meaning I had to make some very hard choices. . .breathing. . .

Poetry and Yoga. . .as inseparable as ocean and sand. Together they create a mirror glass reflecting the enlightenment inside of us. Yoga turns us inward as we discover the graceful flow of our bodies interacting with breath and spirit; poetry channels expression outwards, pouring in the shape of words onto paper. Letters bend as a yoga asana, creating paragraphs with our lives. Feelings unravel in the form of sentences buried deep inside.

Dawn looks forward to dusk. . .resting its enlivened eyes on a paint-brush, a sunset, a head on a yoga mat. The yoga mat is the canvas for many artists unscrewing the lid to the soul jar. . .peering inside and liberating the colors. . .yes, there are still colors we have yet to see. . .time is moved by oceans; sand wishes to become glass again; rebirth; your body paints poetry through asana on a canvas mat; love is just moments away; union.

In a world filled with contradictions, we need steady confusion to assist us in knowing clarity. A light bends into the crevice of a heart-ache. . .our hearts open to the dancing knowledge of expression. We are at the cusp of spiritual revolution in the modern day.

This collection of modern day poetry is testament. It sings of not only Mirabai and Hafiz. . .but Swenson and Rea; it breathes not only of Rumi and Gibran. . .but Folan and Stryker.

This book is a clear signal that forgiveness and compassion are rooted in our souls. . .as deep as the need for survival is the need for creative expression and cooperation. Technology cannot dampen our poetic spirits. Instead we are creatively learning how to use it as a tool to help us express and release what is locked in our muscles and bones. . .through spirit-filled words. With all of your loving kindness and support my initial mission has been accomplished.

Now, the other part of the mission is for this anthology to raise money for the dynamic work of a great non-profit organization called One Common Unity. Ultimately, I hope this book and the subsequent volume, will provide a sustainable source of revenue for the work they have been doing since the year 2000.

One Common Unity supports a movement for peace education and the building of a non-violent culture through music and art. More specifically, they facilitate arts-based health and wellness, conflict resolution, and nonviolence education for inner-city youth.

Spiritual warriors, compassionate renegades, lovers of truth and seekers of wisdom. . .the time is now; let these words breathe through the pores of your skin. Let your mind stir, the hairs on your arms stand, and let this be a reminder that we have not lost our souls.

Regardless of your race, nationality, sexuality, age, class, religion, or gender, there is something in this book for everyone. Read in awe and wonder. . .as I did. . .I hope you do. . .embrace all the magical poetry in this collection. Take it around the world with you and let it serve proof of the modern day poetic soul of humanity.

Your Reflection,

HawaH

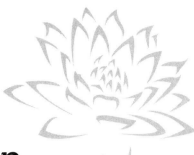

Compassion

Your shoes
Are on my feet
I know now
Why your socks are ripped
The draft moves my heart.

HawaH

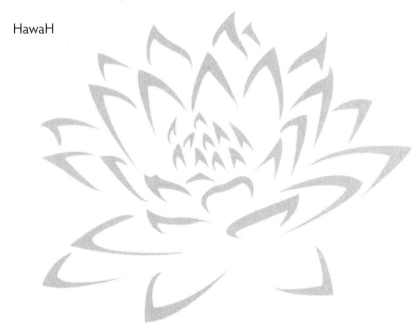

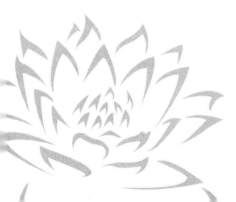

Prasad

That sound you hear?
It's my frozen heart melting.

Bringing each drop to my lips,
I cover my body freely,

wet with your name.
My lips become your lips,

my body your body.
When I take you into me,

the world goes on forever.
I will find peace

in these fragments.
This pain will be the cure.

Prasad: *Sanskrit, literally, "A precious gift." An offering, usually a sweet or some other food, blessed by an enlightened being and given to her/ his followers.*

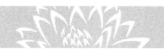

In a Corner of the Body, a Thief Sits Waiting

In a corner of the body,
a thief sits waiting
to steal your affection.
Like a pickpocket in the black market,
he hides in the dark alleys of the body,
but your virtues are a lantern
rooting him out.

Catch a glimpse
as he rounds the corner
hoping to hide in the hip joint.
Watch him fly
as he darts between the shoulder blades,
wedges himself therein.
Marvel as he ducks
under the sacrum, sticks there
like a thumbtack.
Rejoice to see him tumble
headfirst into the pelvic bowl,
jeering as he peers around its rim.

Don't let his alacrity fool you.
He's as slow as what limits you,
holding you back just as much.
Once you catch him with your awareness,
don't throw him into prison.
Don't bind him up in rope.
Rather, hang him out in the light,
and praise him effusively.

For when the chase is over,
he will have taught you
the many secrets of the maze,
and you can start to polish
all those precious gems
he's been guarding.

The Edge

Each time the world
pushes you to the edge
asking of you
more than you can bear,
go ahead anyway
even if—or because—
you're straining against
an invisible net.

Let yourself burst at the seams
until the seams themselves stretch,
and the net tears, floats away
into the nothingness
from which you came.
Who holds the net anyway?

Everything it contains
will come rushing forth.
Embrace it all, and then some.
You'll grow bigger than you ever imagined.

So much I want to say to you, teacher!
But you say: *just live your best life.*
It speaks so much more eloquently
than words.

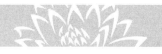

In Me

Once, I was looking for fireflies in the night,
Now, I find all the stars are shining in me.

Once, I was getting lost on the way,
Now, I find all roads joining in me.

Once, long seasons passed in waiting,
Now, all meetings are happening in me.

Once, even the rivers were running dry,
Now, all the oceans are dancing in me.

Once, the leaves of autumn were floating,
Now, a million springs are blooming in me.

Once, each moment seemed full of clamour,
Now, even time has fallen silent in me.

Once, even sparks were missing in life,
Now, a thousand lamps are alight in me.

Once, hands were joined in prayer,
Now, infinite blessings reside in me.

Once, the soil of the heart was parched,
Now, bountiful showers are pouring in me.

Once, the earth was just like a prison,
Now, the boundless sky lives in me.

Timeless Song

In the heart's dawn
rises a sacred song,
filled with your light.
It gently touches
my myriad passions
that bloom into
an ardent love.

This fragrant prayer
floats into clouds
of devotion that
pour down in
the rains of joy,
flowers of tears
at your sacred feet.

Once more the
world rejoices
in the thrill of
a secret love,
a timeless melody,
always ancient,
yet ever-new.

Gratitude for the Mat

I lay you down to greet the sun,
a firm base for my tadasana.
You grab my hands as I bow down,
securing my pose in your grip,
never the first to let go.

As breath stretches limbs,
heavy memories trapped in
cells shed from my skin.
You fold them up in your tight lips,
never to speak of them again.

You are my rock, my roots,
my cradle in Savasana.
You transform from solid to soft,
echoing the process of practice.
Only you witness those sweet divine moments
when tears slip from my face to yours.

A closing OM benediction
soaks into your fibers,
ending our union for now.
I say goodbye with a curl of my fingers
and fasten you up,
hoping to soon meet again.

And so, my loyal friend,
rolled in the corner
like a fresh cut log,
waiting in your quiver to be
unwrapped for worship,
I thank you.

Love Is

Love is an illusion until you can love yourself
in your disappointment,
in your uncertainty,
in a vacuum of nothingness.

Love is moving out of fear of your body, your mind,
your self into the quest of acceptance.

Love is feeling wretched, and knowing it's okay.
love is listening to beads pour;
love is the burble of brooks,
the beat of your heart.

Love is letting yourself be in love,
out of love, tired of love.

Love is all of it because
you and only you,
know the courage it takes
to be in love
with you,

when your body screams,
No.

Seeing Milarepa: a Movie About a Tibetan Saint

It makes me sad to see
pigeons well-fed
by the veiled woman
refusing to share nuts with squirrels

I walk to Cinema Village

Enemies are never ending
popcorn is finite
whispers the ticket taker

Milarepa sought salvation
for vengeance taken
against mind and bone
of those who'd done him harm

He wrote poems
of skillful means
taught compassion served tea
I write notes in the dark

There are lines we can not change
camera angles which test our will
whispers the ticket taker

Broken Glasses

the woman enters yoga
late
shifting to make room
i crush my bifocals
a hundred expletives
upon her banana blonde hair
until i remember
almost dying in the cold
last winter
when a metal beam
fell from a building
crashing against my shadow
we're all vulnerable
without sight improvement technology
my vision's 20/200
it's night
oncoming headlights
shine like mutant fireflies
i lift my shirt and sternum
beaming blurry eyed compassion
at a hundred taxis
at every bone
ever broken
every nuance
ever grasped

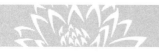

Prayer Without Flowers

O Lord, You gave me a vase
to keep loveliness in.
I have filled and refilled it
my entire life; but every time,
the light within the beauty I have gathered
fades away, leaving fragrant memories
that turn to powder when I handle them.

So now I display Your gift
empty. I admire it simply
for its form and solitude,
and for the way it craves
to be filled.

Exhale

Who dem spirits
you be fighting
when we be making love

How you gonna show me
sun sky rain
not expecting to see

Rainbows
dancing sidewalk
under my feet

Yoga in the afternoon
Sunshine when I look up
The promise of sweetness

you say
No Goddess left behind
I say

I am
you say
like sweet fruit

I say
nobody love you like me
moaning sweet and low

does breath life love
green blue black and yellow
stop

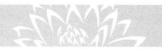

do eyes say
what's read
when you grab hold

You like my potions
love them even
drink them down

Without
question
Or hesitation

Sundials
alabaster
Lapis

Orange Peel
Copal & Myrrh,
Brown sugar & Amber
Honey & Lemongrass

There is a healing
happening
while these things burn

There is a sweet smell
a warmth
emanating throughout

Wide-open spaces
Warm desert breezes
Muladhara to my Sahasrara

Chakras spinning

Inhale
Like a midday breeze
Surrounding you

Getting lost
then
Finding self again

Dropping old memories
I'm placing beautiful things
in the temple

and
it smells like bliss

This exorcism was needed
Space and peace
now

A Daily Practice

Weight on my hands, knees bent,
arms like metal brackets, elbows pointed,
making 90-degree angles of my arms.
If I were stronger I'd lift one knee and balance it
on the table I've made between forearm
and elbow, but with a body not yet
fit after carrying and birthing a third
child, I'd rather assume child's pose—

Arms flung forward, kneeling in surrender.
The teacher says: Fear limits us.
I've been fearful all my life: of elevators, escalators,
flash mobs, planned mobs, on New Year's Eve,
Times Square on a spring day,
streets littered with too many souls,
vultures circling skyscrapers, alligators.

The teacher says: Can you play with fear?
What he means is can you make a space
within your fear for the grace of one breath?
Can you breathe in it, can you breathe through it?
Can you balance it with peace, with hope?
When I taught second graders how
to write poems, I asked them think about hope
and fear. To them, hope was anything
from "hugging my mother" to "having dinner
with my whole family." Fear was more than once
"hearing gun shots on my street when I go
to sleep" and "not passing into the third grade."

I rise up, with shoulders solid as pylons
in the ocean. One knee balances on my forearm.
I lean forward, lifting the other leg. My fear hollows
in the wave of each breath. My fear
like the cicada shells I'd find in springtime:
hard, brown, brittle. I never saw one shed
its shell, never witnessed the change from nymph to adult,
from one way of being to another, but at night
it happened again and again. Moon as witness,
stars as witness. Nothing in this class
is as scary as life. I unbind and emerge. Space
in each breath, opening in the body, the mind,
feet parallel, strong center, palms together. The world
outside, outside. The teacher's voice within: Your
practice begins when you leave this room.

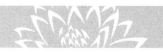

Under Your Very Toes

Along with its fellow planets
Rolling on
In their limitless playground
This bluegreen wonder marble
Lets us in
For a free ride
Turn after turn

We humans
Ego-logically shortsighted
Trotting about, unaware
Tickling and tingling the earth-skin
As we go

Stop!
And listen
And listen again
Under your very toes

(Can you hear the giggle?)

Limbs

(Nidra)
I dream of nothing
but this one moment
when all of me
has expanded
beyond recognition

(Tapas)
I crave sugar
when I've lost sweetness,
but dare not medicate
such a wound with a Band-Aid.
Rather, I grow from within
the nectar of seekers.

(Prana)
I am ever moving wind
that makes the music of chimes
and the rustle of leaves,
lest you forget
I am ever with you
dancing upon your tongue.

(Transformation)
This playground is lonely
without the knowledge of laughter.

(Natarajasana)
The body
she remembers
all the toils of the mind,
war crimes,
humanity industrialized.
Still, she finds balance.
But she's a victim
of the injustice of time.
Behold her for a moment
and with the blinking of eyes
she falls into the next.
Pray love embraces her
and she escapes
the gripings of death.

Repetition of steps:
the deception of stress
revealing all of man's neglect
with untamed beatings of the chest.
Still, what joy
to be gifted with such a mess.
What life to live
with the promise
of no regrets.

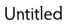

Untitled

with a feather
the universe is untangled

Sadhana

I have crossed this
Earth as
a student and didn't see you
as a teacher
and could not conjure you
I lifted stone
and stepped in soil
I have chanted your name
and breathed the techniques
practiced the particulars
that are mentioned in texts
representing you
I have found these beautiful stones
placed them on the altar and dedicated
it all to you
I have picked up fallen petals
and plucked new ones
all for you
I watch the moon
and feel the breath and a mudra
one that tastes you
I have been tired and not rested
and I've fallen in the darkest depth
I have danced and sat
been brave and a coward
have stolen and given my all
Animals, children and people have loved me
I have believed them all
and none of them
these years seem so short
a yesterday, at best

God, Whispering

Inside of
one snowflake
there is a
waterfall
where God is
taking a bath.

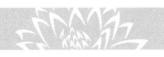

Solid

In the dawn of summer,
I slipped out from the cabin
Unleashing myself, alone into the unknown
Crept free from any tracings of my whereabouts.
Skipped along, downhill upon a dirt path
Stenciled by the rising Sun
Matching breath with step
Hopping from one stone to the next
Dancing round trees agilely
While fire breathing
The ambrosial scents of morning
Honoring everything divine—within this forest and I

Trekking deeper until a cool shoreline met my toes.
From my palms, I took a sip, and as if
Some potion had ignited the process of absorption
Through my bloodstream,
Some power overcame me

Scaling boulders to their peaks—I was a leaping lioness
Paused by a pose in sudden silence—and embrace of ego
Orange illuminations refracted around my entire being
The lake's surface mirrored life at large in this moment's glow
And for one split second the world slowed
Then stopped spinning.

I was locked—onto this rock—as if we had been slit apart
          thousands of years ago.

Even after all our time being worn and weathered
We reunited—and meshed perfectly
Like crystallized puzzle pieces
We were one.

Surrender

And then comes the moment of surrender,
not because it's the only thing I can do but because
it's the only thing I want to do. . .
It is in this state of surrender where transformation lies
and patiently waits for my arrival as a holy guest once more

Face down
bowing at your feet
in full pranam
as light surrenders to dark,
day to night
unabashedly
holding nothing back

There is nothing more to hold onto

My whole body weeping
soaked and drenched in tears
bursting at the seams with
doubt and confusion
take all of me
take me, I'm yours
I must die to myself
and love yet again.

Yogini on Fire

naked
in my truth
raw in my honesty
nothing to hide
no shame to wear
anything can happen now
in the womb of Kali
swallowed whole
undeniable power of Her swift sword
She holds me
it's total fierce love

clear
the arrow knows the way
intrepid path
lineages of Grace
rivers of revelation
Saraswati flows
insight surges
dances
On the tip
of the poet's tongue
on the edge of immortality

radiant
lotus rising
great ocean of compassion
giving birth to the moonlit glow
softening my edges
like the intimate caress of a lover
in the middle of the night
Her lotus eyes
Lakshmi blazing
in the pure heart fire
the nectar of my soul

Love Raid

You are Perfect
You are Grace
You are Love

Everything about you is perfection becoming more perfect
There's no end to your perfection
You Are That
You are the Great Expanse
Of Perfection becoming more perfect

How can Grace fall from Grace?
You cannot fall from Grace
You are Grace
Grace falls as Grace
It's too big of a burden
To carry around
Thinking that you've fallen from Grace

She has not deserted you
She has not cast you out
You cannot catch her
She never ran away from you
She is You

And when She does fall
It's just like perfect ripe fruit
In the flow of gravity
Cracking open on this earth
Offering nourishment to all

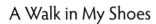

A Walk in My Shoes

You see me as fat
I walk with the notion that one more bite will fill this emptiness
inside me

You see me as an addict
I walk with years of physical abuse that can only be forgotten when
I swallow this pill or take that drink

You see me as a rebellious teen
I walk with constant ridicule and rejection

You see scars
I walk with reminders of the days when no one paid attention

You see me as 'perfect'
I walk with fear of never being good enough

You see me as a Yogi
I walk in constant refinement

You see.
I am.

Ethos

The brown paper napkins are stacked,
the wooden floor gleams and the sconces flicker.
The sun filters through the French doors
with the white billows;
cat comes in first always languid and light,
while placid cows breathe and feel the spirals of sensation,
as we descend into plank, breath lifts us into cobra
and soon jubilant hips angle into dog. . .
gurus, prophets, sages, mystics for a moment,
we climb into warriors, letting go of all the doing,
dropping it softly as knees fall into child's pose,
sillystupid at our best with our applesauce crossed legs
holding hula hoops under our arms,
our shoulders melting like vegan butter—
Soon the foundation of oceanic rhythms give way,
releasing the I, the WE, and ever present me, me, me—
Our bodies, clay pots are thrown with each breath,
glazed with each movement, ready as the heat rises,
we glisten with each new firing,
as our vessels' impurities bead and drop,
we leave, we grow into
good enough mothers,
compassionate enough fathers,
smart enough sisters and strong enough brothers.
Taller, we begin again. . .
ready to share a little more,
ready to fight a little less.

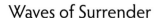

Waves of Surrender

It is never as expected
this breath
that movement
something that awakens
the underlying current
that rocks my soul, my bones, my child-seeds
and brings my attention to a peak
from which I can see
the stars, the rivers,
and the darkness.

There is a symphony
that plays within our bodies
Igniting the particles around me
and sparking the light
within you.

The stars join in
playing their instruments
and the music is heard
in the still spaces
between the Beatles
and the foot traffic below.

It is never as expected
the student finding the teacher
The teacher bowing to become
the student
The universe exhaling
to remind us
that it is
okay
to let go.

Full Cambodia Bellies

Your lips part gently, revealing surprisingly white teeth.
I scoop a heap of white rice as my eyes recognize
the tiny black specks sprinkled through as the aftermath
of a hungry mouse's feast.
Guilt pinches the passage in which my breath flows
causing an unfamiliar gasp,
but your eyes remain bright as the sun
that drenches the longing earth.
The sounds of your slurping ring
appreciation through the polluted air
and for a moment it feels clean.
You feel clean,
despite the immortal dirt embedded in your cuticles
reminding me of how those little fingers
once scavenged for recyclables
in football fields of people's unwanted particles.
And for a moment a wave of grace fills my lungs
as I swallow the beauty before me.
How your light was never dimmed baffles me
but I then remember
love can thrive in even the dirtiest conditions.
Even in piles of trash.
Even in piles of hate.
Even in piles of Genocide.
Love can exist like the lone lotus
in the wretched filth infested swamp.
With no effort.
With no pain.
It simply thrives.
You finish your soupy rice concoction
as your belly resonates a satiated glow
and I know you are fulfilled.

Sweet India

I long to take sweet breaths of wisdom,
masked by the funk of dirt roads paved with cow manure.
If I get still enough I can smell it,
despite the fact that I am half way across the world.

It followed me lovingly as I traveled your earth,
embedded with tracks of many footprints searching.
They are always searching.

I want to desperately feel the heat of your sun
scorch the accidentally exposed strip of skin
on my embarrassed shoulder.

I want to feel the splatters of mud slap my calf
as it is flung from my flip flops.
But I am afraid.

For if I leave the neatly nestled confines of my country
in search of a truth I can so easily see
when I am feet away from the majesty of the Himalayas,
plunging my toes in the courage of the Ganga,
I know I may never return.

But then I remember what you helped to reveal
is neatly nestled in the meadows and fields of my heart,
embedded in the clouds and oceans that are my soul.
It is the very fabric of my breath
and the vision I see when my eyes are clear.

And I can feel that anywhere.
But with your help it surely is the sweetest.

Equinox

Moons take our measure,
suns pour over, tides flow within,
air moves through—

sometimes we fall,
sometimes fly,
sometimes are hollow,
sometimes fill our skins.

No one can say which is the birthing day
or name the day of our dying
when the sky is a door, open.

Awaken

I.

We are in the wake of a great shifting,
awaken

II.

You better free your mind
before they illegalize thought

there's a war going on

the first casualty was truth
and it's inside you

the universe is counting on our belief
that faith is more powerful than fear
and that in this shifting moment
we'll all remember why we're here

III.

Because
Love is God
and God is Truth
and Truth is You
and You are Me
and I am Everything
and Everything is Nothing
and Nothing is the Birthplace of Creation
and transformation is possible
and you are proof

and the most powerful tool in the hands of the oppressor
is what's inside our heads

and the most dangerous weapon to combat the deception
lives inside our chests
hold a mirror to your heart
what does it reflect?
what will be the message
of the legacy we've left?

IV.

We were born right now for a reason
we can be whatever we give ourselves the power to be

and right now we need dream-weavers,
bridge-builders, truth-sayers,
light-bearers, food-growers,
wound-healers, trail-blazers,
life-lovers, peace-makers

give what you most deeply desire to give
every moment you are choosing to live
or are you waiting

why would a flower hesitate to open?
now is the only moment
rain drop let go
become the ocean
possibility is as wide
as the space we create to hold it

V.

the stars have spent lifetimes
trying to reach us with the message
that our light can inspire solar systems if we let it
shine like the moon's reflection

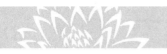

of her suns and daughters
great great great grandmothers and fathers
foretold this time of great blessing and slaughter
when we'd decide between drought
and drowning in water

or rising like mist from toxic streams
with dreams of becoming rainwater
that falls pure to the earth
to quench the thirst we'd forgotten
was the reason we struggle in
this web that we're caught in

is not a trap
but an intricate pattern
like a labyrinth, a snowflake
or crystal of water

or the concentric rings of a tree
that still makes a sound
long after its fallen
in a forest that lived
even if no one saw it
and fed the world its breath
whether or not we applauded
one hand clapping sounds a lot like
the rhythm we lost in
generations who sang
even as they departed

we paved concrete
over the pores of the earth
to make our lives harder
and built buildings to scrape skies
trying to get closer to God
but moved farther

from the source that birthed
the first light in the darkness

we stole from our mother
and we continue to rob her
for diamonds and gold
and our ancestors' bones
disappeared from their coffins

turned hollow
so they could fly
with the weight of the fodder
on her wings she has
dust inside her brain
and got caught up
thinking pain was her fate
but this is what you said that you wanted

whether we knew it or not
the universe responded
to every vision and image
and nightmare we've thought of

our words are like bullets
and we call the shots
by their names
and they come running
with gifts in their pockets

impressions of lessons of
the stories
life taught us
that our dreams are impossible
so we keep them in closets
and now we stand at the doorway

in the hallway
life brought us
to this cross roads
of lost hope and undeniable promise
where we choose between paths
beyond rightness or wrongness
that will lead to the brink
of the planet's exhaustion
or the age of compassion
where the meek become strongest
and reinherit the earth
and redefine progress

VI.

don't be scared of the spark
in the spell of great darkness
or afraid of the light
in the moment of dawning
or the heights you will reach
when you rise to your calling
and release all your rain
call it flying
or falling
let go of your wanting
and give into your longing
to live free of possessions
and full of belonging
to the intricate infinity
we're all a part of
the web that you wove
in a dream you'd forgotten
was the Creator awaking
into your conscious
condensation of vapor
into a droplet of water

Tajeme

You could hear the sound
Of the steel against his body

Still

Ricocheting throughout our ribcages
The day we lost him
Our hearts
Excavated out
Left a hollow impression of life
Like the 6-foot hole in the ground they put him in

Our spirits bent with the weight of his casket
The winter threatened to crack us open like the autopsy report
And the newspaper clippings
I'm sure his mama cut and saved
For fear of missing him too much

We pulled from the sky
And collected puddles on our collarbones

She tucked herself into the folded edges of her son's eulogy

We all walked around like question marks for weeks
Backs so round
Knees threatened to buckle

It's a dangerous place to find yourself
Angry
With no answers

With no solid ground to stand on
We were floating sage
No lights on this stage
These weren't actors

On the block they killed him
The cops laughed at us
For burning candles
And I wondered who had taken their humanity
Not even Hollywood could have conjured up this sickness

I wondered about the preacher
Whose voice riddled Bible passages throughout the funeral
And compared his love to the love of Jesus
But misrepresented this poet
Who wrote proses for the universe's stolen moments
When he asked all the men
To either unwrap their heads
Or leave God's home
With their anger still woven within them

His God doesn't have arms wide enough
For the Rastas
The Muslims
The Jews
The mourners
Tajeme's friends
Who pay homage by covering their entry way to heaven
People have a million ways of disrespecting life
You don't have to pull a trigger

But somebody shot him
Multiple times in the chest and arms
To pay back someone's miscalculated footing
We don't know what happened
All we know is that the NYPD sees
Black
Male
6 feet 5 inches
Gun violence

And I have to laugh to keep from crying
Think of Chris Rock when I think of bullet prices
Statistics can feel like sugar in the sun
To an already open sore
25 cent for a round of bullets?
It costs less than a penny to kill a human
A brother
An artist
A giver
A believer of life
A dreamer of the impossible
A carpenter
Who painted colorful walls on his days off
For disabled children
And made their living in a room possible

A magic maker
Who grabbed your hands
And made the impractical, toss-able
An open door
The Cheshire Cat's smile on a broke journey
The wind against your back
If you were hauling ass
Or moving
From this side to the other side Brooklyn

It didn't matter

His hands were big
Curled into a fist his heart was bigger
A sunlight keeper
We know the stars whitewashed his soul
on his way to the creator
And left no sign of gun powder
Or the smell of fear on his killers

A penny for a death can cost a fortune to your spirit
And all this violence paints, is a people not worth living
In a culture that only incarcerates the darkest children

My heart is bleeding from the cold slap insult of ignorance
A post-traumatic slave syndrome
Where we settle arguments
Like slave keepers

Who planted these seeds?
And who's gonna reap them?

Television already brainwashing our self image
Got us scared of looking deep
Cause we're scared of the dark

And black is bad

And the depth of our soul is a black hole
That might stretch time and reinvent the unknown
From impossible to unbelievable

So we tell white lies to our inner children

And hope the root cause of this tree
Is strong enough to keep this landslide from slipping
But we're dripping more than sweat
Playing the wrong hand we've been given

Even though none of us can believe it

My brother's death is not a coincidence
It's a catalyst for reconfiguring
The sacred geometry of living

Bloom

Never forget that you longed for this.
Even as you begin to complicate your contemplations,
considering the many sub-standard sensations
existence tends to thrust upon one
in those withering, early hours of the morn'
when even Marigolds,
amidst the overwhelming fields
of Springtime's fingerpaints,
occasionally entertain the notion of "calling in sick",
yet somehow
still manage
to rise to the occasion
and bloom.

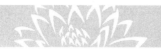

Love

All love in compassion
All compassion in understanding
All understanding in letting go
All letting go in love

Karma Yoga

i must learn to give myself away
as effortlessly as the wind blows across the reeds
or as carefree as dandelions lose their parts
to the soft gentle tearing of those gathering in the crisp
white-yellow fields

if i act, it must be for the good of others
not the intention of recognition or the glorification of self

if i move, it must be to become the swift feet of others
not to climb the self-deluded ladder of success

if i believe, it must be to have faith
to meditate upon God and what is good

if i am to question, it must be to ask how can i help

if i think, it must be to think of others,
not to think of myself

if i am to be at all
it is to be for you

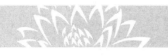

Relinquishment

If all this plenty my eyes survey shall pass away
The tribes and familial bonds too,
Little ones running in the sand boxes,
And lunches packed,
If in some other life I will forget this broken bread?

If I forget my tears shed, and my broken heart,
Or the Thanksgiving Day dinners,
Or walking hand in hand,
If in my age as my eyes start to snap shut
Like unpolished oyster shells

And I am left open and alone,
And not I, even I, will remain upon this earth
Except in spirit and bones,

Love between husband and wife will extinguish
Beneath the big moon's rising and setting
Against the ocean waves,

What stays, my dear,
What is the word forever for?

The Idea I Used to Believe In

This morning has that certain texture.
The kind where everything Belongs

The only thing out of place now
Would be the idea I used to believe in

The one that goes:
I know that formula
for making everything belong,
I've seen it used a hundred times

Too bad it doesn't work that way

This morning is more like pouring infinity
Into a paper cup

Spilling everywhere,
Knocking over everything

The whole time laughing
At this most beautiful
Intoxicating mess

Water*asana*

I am liquid
    hips pouring
        a fluid spine
            while shoulders
                cascade down
                    a flowing waterfall
                        this buoyant body's
                            carving canyons
                        etching out my history
                  in supplicate sandstone
                mellifluous sounds resonate
            from this splashing
        two arms trickle
            towards the earth
                out of a pool of muscle, bone
                    as my ocean of breath, dulcet
                        laps at the shores of simple
                              consciousness

A Modern Devotion

Circumnavigating mountains,
we're the knees of pilgrims.

Bent.
Prostrate.

Kiss the gravel
and forget you know my name
because,
You are my name.

Feel the crease
the back of the knee,
aching tendons stuck
in a quicksand spiral
a temporary insanity stretch
towards the divine.
Polar caps and opposites attract.

We lay our palms.
Allow fingerprints to caress
the earth with our identity
Become the soil as flecks
Of our skin join specks of our dirt.

Light at the end of the horizon
Lingers on forehead
reminding
the final part of our period of time
is just ash trays and coffee grinds.
A lifetime of:
inhaling burnt tobacco
and
ingesting burnt beans

A spine curls into dust.
Supple.
As we always knew we were intended to be.

And so, we go.
Our footsteps arching pathways
tread towards center, we flow

As a Core,
Heart,
Mind's eye blinks

A flutter in the flame like tissue paper candles quiver

You lag behind.
Slumped shoulders tell your story
You place your blame.
A golden star sticker upon my chest, Scarlet A
You place me.
Our journey.
Twisting the Mason jar's lid. . .sealed.

Away.
We've floated here before
So the instinct says.

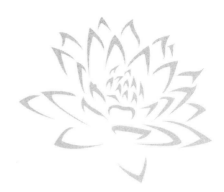

Desire

I was born searching for memories
As an experience desires to be remembered
As a song desires to be heard

HawaH

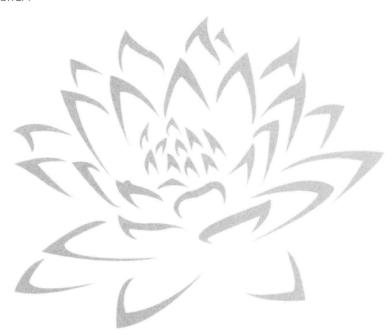

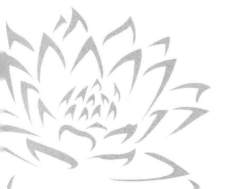

I Am Here For You

Always—I am here for you
Escape your busy life
Don't talk. . .just join me
Savor my understanding, and my love

Arouse your senses
Taste the fruit of my alluring gift
Or indulge completely
In the vast orchard, of life's sacred passion

Smell the blossoms of desire
Be with me—feel what is in your heart
You are not that busy. . .
You are never—too busy for me

Come with me, pick the whole fruit
And sit under the tree of life
Surrender completely
As love, is well spent with me

Tomorrow is too late
I will be gone!

Always I am here for you. . .
Yet sadly, always I must leave
Eternity—is the time we spend together

Forever and always. . .I am here for you
This moment loves you!

You Will Find It

Beyond the teasing minds—of yesterday's faults
Beyond the purity of tomorrow's reflection

Beyond the rain—that has not yet fallen
Beyond the fluffy clouds, still sleeping in the ocean

Beyond the future dreams—of a distant society
Beyond this mirage of creation

Find the dawn of energy. . .
waiting patiently for you to awake
Limits are only—for those who believe

Tell Me How

I am not impressed
With the type of car you drive
    Tell me how you...
      Roll on your own two feet

I am not impressed
With how much money you have
    Tell me how you...
      Find riches in simplicity

I am not impressed
With your popular friends and spouse
    Tell me how you...
      Have your own game too

I am not impressed
With your cool—exclusive groups
    Tell me how you...
      Stand alone, as spirit of conviction

I am not impressed
With your trophy, stuffed animals
    Tell me how you...
      Find strength in preservation of life

I am not impressed
With your fancy commercial foods
    Tell me how you...
      Find heaven in a leaf of kale

I am not impressed
With polished words and stylish clothes
    Tell me how you...
      See beauty in the heart and soul

I am not impressed
With your political party
    Tell me how you. . .
        Resist team play and peer pressure

I am not impressed
With your boxed religious speeches
    Tell me how you. . .
        See all ways, as different paths up the mountain

I am not impressed
With your degrees and education
    Tell me how you. . .
        Learned from oceans and mountains

I am not impressed
With what you think you know
    Tell me how you. . .
        Aspire to learn from others

I am not impressed
With your number of lovers
    Tell me how you. . .
        Hug the homeless and love kindness

I am not impressed. . .
With most of the usual things
    Tell me how you. . .
        Ride rainbows and water dreams

    Tell me how you. . .
        Stay Human
            Please do.

Restoration

There was a moment in the parking lot
after no-breath-chest-jammed conniption
in a grey cubicle farm. My friend thought
I was dying. She said women have different
symptoms for heart
attacks.

Later, the Iyengar physical therapist taught me
with a simple bolster on the smooth flat
coolness of the floor
how to open my heart.
Restoration
came
in waves.

They say the heart's our center,
our portal down into the
core of the planet. I had been running
so long, full out, angry,
it took an inner earthquake
to shake me down
past the lines of fault
to the sweet, round curve
of the planet. Now I am
nestled and stretched
on the wake of her, arms out
flying into spaces
so wide and even.
This is the generous breath
now, in the core of me,
a tender touch,
still and curving,
open and spacious:
planetary restoration.

Solidify Before You Fly

Seriously,

Unraveling this mystery of me
Is a truthful undertaking
Rising to my root
To travel the core beyond my creation

Nothing to lose but the way that I was
Lying dead on the road ahead

Symbolically—ironically
I seem a renegade rafter
In a time long last and before

Cutting between
The self sovereign
And the self less necessity

Tasting my tongue still to touch on the tissues of matter
Solidify before I fly

Rooting to rise
To ripen before
I fall

Becoming the seed of life sustaining it all

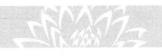

In the Moment

laughter and love
love and laughter
if that is your NOW
who cares what comes after

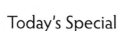

Today's Special

MENU:

Down economies
Wars and Recessions
Environmental disasters
Global injustice

Uncertain future
Human minds busier
Preoccupied with
Devastation or Preservation

Nonetheless
Today's special is:

An unblemished sky
Hosting a golden light ball of
Rounded perfection

Its stillness a
Dynamic reflection
Served on a dancing ocean

Waves born and die
Piano, crescendo, forte
Crushing refrains of water

Meeting the earth.

A Limerick on Non-Attachment

There was a young man from Rathmines
Who thought Limericks should have just two lines

Untitled

It's the dirty of first snow melting.
Dead trees that shimmer with cold manifested,
Attached and holding on like the hair on his chest.
Log homes, layered clothes.
My things still smell of woodsmoke and wine,
Scent-wrapped,
Like the heat did my body on a brown tweed couch
In the basement of a tired town.

He held himself tightly,
And despite my mind wanting,
I didn't move to make him stop.

So he did.

That's when I found lines along muscles
and shared space between thoughts.
That's maybe even why.
It's funny how strength and pain occupies the same,
In tissue and backbones that carry each other.
In touching one, I felt the other.

We let go like this;
Like words on the wings of paper aeroplanes,
lost in the wind.

The pages unfold to blankness,
drift to settle against my skin.
I left them unwritten.
Stayed respectful of the clean unseen,
At peace in the ice or the fire.
There's much to be said for the present's desire—
Nothing more, nothing less.

Although, truth be told, it was hard to go,

To pass on the act of intervening.

So I thought of all the love I have,
and sent some words to give it back,
and sighed the happy kind for my sweet and simple life.

I'm still,
Alone,
And everything is beautiful.

Fields of Roses

In Tree Pose
I stand
grounded, tall, secure
for you

In Toe Stand
I give my all
with full attention and will
for your peace

In Spinal Twist
my eyes turn to see
you run freely
in fields of roses

And in that last Savasana
as I close my eyes
I surrender to the silence—
the restful place of freedom
where roses bloom

Body's Melody

Every part of our body,
An indispensable detail in our posture

Our posture, the playing of our instrument
Its melody, the song of our inner self

Our inner self, the source of our art
In our source, a masterpiece

Thank you, body,
every part.

Lord of the Fishes

When does the connection between heart
    and voice become solid
yellow line, not broken, how long
    have I shied away
from the pose of the fish
    or buried my voice
in the murky pond of shame?
    Midweek
Lynnette tells me after class,
    Thursday used to
be her drinking night, now
    it's her yoga night.
How long for these shifts,
    all these years
I had lied to protect whom?
    Me, my family,
from what. . .the fear that no one
    would stop
and listen to me, the way Matsya
    hooked
by Lord Shiva's story, stayed,
    the way these brave women
return week after week,
    why did I not think
those I loved would open their hearts
    to me,
Or why do any of us doubt
    the safe net
of another's heart, the power
    of our own?

Drishte

This morning, rain again,
all that back and forth
The windshield wipers
give momentary relief

from the inevitable.
I watch the headlights
on the other side
of the divided highway,

remembering how sometimes
the other drivers
would flick them off and on
in warning

speed trap. Slow down
and I can't
help but thinking
how these small unspoken flickers

could be like fireflies
signaling their presence
to each other
and how when we were younger

we collected them in a jar
as if we couldn't see the light
in our own eyes,
like how you look at me

when I am walking towards you
in the airport,
two blue suns, arms
rays

When is something what it is
and when is it something else.

Shraddha

If nothing is yours,
nothing can be taken from you,

but how easy to want,
how easy to say, mine.

How not to hold your hand,
or fold my body into yours

thinking, yes, you will always be here
when earlier we had seen the dead trees.

An entire landscape changed, gone.
"Pine beetles," Flavien explains,

"this happens every fifty years," he says
as he drives us around the preserve.

At Caracol Fredy tells us
blue morpho butterflies are fallen warriors

returned to us
and Mayan astrologers would count the stars

every night watching
for new light—

an ancestor
who finally arrived in heaven.

All the things we do to acknowledge
something greater.

Our first night here
we felt our way back

through the dark to our cottage
when the generator went out.

No electricity, no ancestors,
only the two of us moving closer

and closer to
what we think we know.

The Meaning of Life—Who Cares?

According to the ancient Yoga sages
Questioning the meaning of life
While living
Is like questioning the meaning of a roller coaster
In the middle of a roller coaster ride.

Or, like questioning the meaning of love
In the middle of lovemaking.

Who cares when something is so amazing?

The amazement IS the meaning.
The amazement IS the ultimate reality.
The amazement IS the life-force of the universe
All around us and within us
Far beyond our ability
To absorb or comprehend.

The amazement IS what some call God
And the ancient sages called Brahman.

In the midst of the ups and downs
Of life and love
Just relax, breathe deeply
And experience the infinite thrill
of the amazing ride.

Silence

Silence is the Roar of the Universe.
Emptiness is the Fullness of the Grand Canyon.
Nothingness is Always Abundance.
Boredom is Always an Invitation to Amazement.
Silence is the Roar of the Universe.

Yoga Tennis

Yoga has transformed my tennis
Like it has transformed everything else.

From the Sutra
I learned to focus on the ball
With single-pointed concentration
To the exclusion of all distractions.

From the Gita
I learned to play hard
Like Arjuna the Warrior
While detaching my ego from the results.

From the Upanishads
I learned cosmic exultation
That all these diverse molecules
Can do all these wondrous things together.

I no longer throw my racket
When I miss an easy shot.
I no longer stay depressed for days
After losing a tough match.

The only problem is
Today I was beaten badly
Because I was distracted
Writing this poem in my head
While I played.

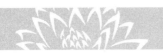

Stillness

The more still we become
the more we descend from our
crystal imaginings
our man-made mirrors
sink into the tender
ferocious efficiency
of the seed

our fleshy density
our tiny eternity
the murmur
underground
pregnant to bursting

no noise
only sound

I Must Talk with Things Falling Away

To straighten your shoulders
In a way that rotates your arms forward
Into the socket. At first it will seem as if you
Are pushing out your chest in a comical
Way or as if you are against the wall
Of a firing squad. Your palms will naturally
Roll forward and open like a flower petal
It is awkward but how things are meant to be
You've grown weary, bending over, hushing
At your desk. Bring the tops of your legs
To attention, feel your knees as they rise
Then straighten and push back your thighs
As if you are holding back a tidal wave
Or a mountain. Tuck your bottom under
Yourself like you aim to sit down but stop
Just before making the decision to do so.
Shrug your shoulders to open up your neck
Turn your chin a little upwards toward
A spot on the wall in front of you, pick
A focus point to stare at but not to sink into.
Spread all ten of your toes and really let your feet
Settle into the earth below as if they were
Homesteading. Now rise above any poses
Or postures or effort or sight or worries you
May have and listen. Just listen. Be quiet
And see what your body comes up with.

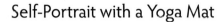

Self-Portrait with a Yoga Mat

I hide behind it, the black, thick
Rubber, soaked with sweat and promise
And intentions, the same every time I unroll
It and start in on the Sun Salutations and the
Series B routines, rituals, prayers.

I do not know who I discovered
Here on the dark
Raft in the middle of this ocean,
Or even what brought me here, one Christmas
When our niece was staying with us following
Her parents' divorce when her father did not want
Her and turned his truck away at the proposed
Pick up time.

I looked at her brown eyes
And freckles and thought of shopping, something
We both hate and then I smiled and said yoga
And so we went.

We struggled to hear the teacher
I tried not to compare it with pilates, my first love
But eventually it came out that yoga was not even
A close second. It was as if I had always done this
Bending and stretching, as if it was what my body
Needed to do, as it furled head-on into the crouching
Spine of the dreaded middle ages.

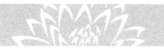

Untitled

The storm is inside my mind,
clouds keep coming.

Static fields dull me,
electric wires are numbing.

I see the sun rising,
a new dawn is here.

I see beauty,
she's standing near.

The water will rise,
I've been swimming for years.

I cleanse myself,
with my own tears.

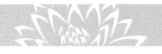

Lessons from my Son

I thought I knew it all
        Then you were born.

You touched my soul to no end
        Your cries burrowed a well
            Stirred my consciousness
                Awakened my humility
A collaboration of love and labor in its purest form.

I see my reflection in your brilliance and turbulence
        Opportunities to heal past wounds
        Nurture vital needs
            Make dreams come true.

You have so much to teach me
        I am ready to learn.

Too Busy to Relax

Too busy to relax they say
Complaints, excuses everyday
They sound so weak, so stressed, so tired
A mundane world in which they're mired
No time to sit and just be quiet
Their mind's a rush of thoughts, a riot
No chance they have to hear the sound
Of nature's wonder all around
Of birds and trees and clouds and air
Too much work, it's just not fair
This really seems quite sad to me
So much to do, no time to be.

Breathe I say and move a bit
Then after that we can just sit
And watch the world at its own pace
There is no rush, it's not a race
And if it were, what is the goal?
Where are you going mind, body, soul?

Too busy to relax I hear
These words seem like they're based in fear
Tired, weak and too much stress
How did our lives turn such a mess?
We don't need to look above
To find a place that's based in love
Turn instead and look within
Find your self, it is no sin
Forgive, let go, open your heart
It is the only place to start
Think on that and you might find
Throughout your life you have been blind.

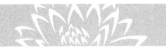
Breathe I say and move some more
Run, walk, jump, stretch on the floor
Move your body, get up and go
Feel the energy, let it flow
Don't get caught in negative
Habits that won't let you live?

Too busy to relax? Not true!
This hoax must end, it starts with you
If all you do is just the same
You never will escape this game
Do something new, do something Zen
Begin right now, not 'if' or 'when'
Do one thing different, or two, or five
Change how you live, become alive
Do or do not, there is no try
Step off the cliff and start to fly
Begin with this, you won't go wrong
Remember to breathe, deep and long.

Autobiography

A wind lifts these pages
Carries them like a fleet of magic carpets
Through the open window.
You've caught one in your hand.
Read it to me.
Tell me who I am.

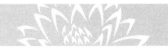

Crescent Moon Pose

This skin holds a universe within
Worlds of star-pocked blackness,
Darkness deeper than eternal oceans.
Between my bones, symphonies sing,
Planets sigh out majestic melodies.
Every vein in me – a Rio Grande all its own.
My lungs, each one a rain forest,
And in my rib cage,
The panting breath of creation,
The desire to live longer than time,
To know the secret
Wrapped in every star.

Absolute

You bit on the
tip of my nose,
Sensuously,
(A throw back
to our animal past!)
Rubbed your nose,
On mine, giving me
A very intimate,
primitive, sensation.
Pecked my lips
affectionately
like a lovelorn
female magpie,
Seeing itself in a mirror.
Filled wine in
your mouth,
and sloshed your
wet full lips over
my taut male nipples.
Bit my ear lobes
till it transmitted waves
of pleasure strikes,
sending lightening sparks
to the primordial depths
of my Mooladhara.
Drove your cruel
long nails
deep in to my back,
till it drew blood.
I was with you
all the while.

But I wasn't
distracted,
My tranquil mind
was in
union with the
Absolute.
and I was possessed by
the consciousness,
Absolute.
And it dawned
on me:
each one of your sensuous
touches was a
glimpse of the
Absolute,
though transient,
like a flash
in the darkness.
So I hold your hands
lovingly, in companionship,
as we complement
each other.
Together we contemplate on
The Sahasrarapadma.
the effulgence eternal
that dispels all darkness.

Poem for an Opening

A yogi sees flowing water
And her heart stretches open
To greet this liquid joy

Then inwardly, she questions
Shall I be flowing water
Or a heart that's soft and moist

Suddenly she sees
That even such reverie
Is too much weight to carry

So she steps away
From all thoughts of beauty
And becomes completely free

Then, very quietly
She enters into the whole of herself
Like a breath

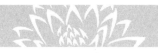

Untitled

Unimaginable Gifts
of such vast quantity
and exquisite, sublime Beauty
Raining down upon our heads
and falling into our hands.
So much that we become numb
and mistake it for Suffering.

Every sound
a signal,
NOW.
Come back to now.
Every crash of the waves,
Every sigh of the wind,
Bird song, leaves rustle.
Scratching of neighbors' feet,
Rustle of cloth,
Creak of chair,
It all says
NOW.
Come Back
to the Silence. . .
Infinite Eternal Silence
the origin of everything

Stay with me a little bit longer
We have come this far together
Hand in hand
two orphans
Innocent and inexperienced
Caught in the role of teachers and leaders
We didn't know it was impossible
So we did it.

nu-wa

a new—nu nu—nu-wa
a new day begins
nature suck and nature splash
a new dawning of a new horrizon
i breathee—you breathee—we breathee—ahhhhhh—

vertical lines and horizontal planes
princess of the sky—protector
a new—new—wa—a nu—wa —wa
shadows dance in the sunlight
triangles float amid cubes and cones
a new—new—nu —a new day dawns

clear—air—energy bright
a nu—new day—a nu—wa—wa

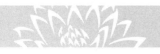
Stealing Angels

This washcloth is a bunched flower
Of cotton turning to silk by the dipping
Under the silver faucet.

Folds of forgotten robes, Turin shrouds
All, forms its blossoms, wet petal by

Petal—
Rain water holy in a basin of glass. . .

Music wells, the songs of souls, names
In our systems, an on-call universe. . .

I can't remember all of them, angel
Thief in my wordy religion, but
The scripture's

Leaves, page after page, pours the faces
From paint—
So many bathed

Bodies, such consoling love, simple
In this kingdom of sighing skin, these
Cathedral cell vessels.

In the end bells & candles give permission
And there is not at all any theft—

Angels of memory, known, unknown,
Heaven hinting, roomfuls of views
Through you and through you. . .

This cloth is the touch of all of that:
Behold the held.

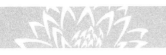

Therefore,
do not be afraid
to let down your guard and relax with others.
Teach others they are not scary
by not being afraid of them.
In this way, they will learn to look out
from their own gentleness
to the gentleness in others.

Your 1st Assignment

Willingly listen inwardly for the voice of your inner Teacher
and learn, be assured, and know
that you can relax inside now and rest,
for you are safe and far from danger.

There is no hurry, walk easy,
but use your time intelligently.
Eagerly want and gladly accept the inner Guide.
Desire, listen for, welcome and embrace
your communion with Me.

This is what you used to refer to as "my little voice."
This is your intuitive knowing,
your contact with Me,
and should be considered quite distinct
from any feelings of guilt.

Listen to your wee little voice,
and let what was temporarily smothered
come to the surface to re-emerge with renewed strength.

Your first assignment is to discover what you want.
Clarify your deepest longings.
Clarify what's important.
Discover this for yourself by listening inwardly.
Simply become quiet and still,
then gently pay attention, watch, listen,
as your deepest motivations
float into your conscious awareness.

Take Another Look

One of the most important things
is to clarify
to yourself
what's important
to you.

What are you really after?
What do you really want?
For understand, there is something that you want,
something you desire deeply.
You are not directionless and without rudder.

But understand also,
the path you have chosen
and the path you are walking,
is the mirror image of what you think important.
Are you following this?

What you are doing
bears witness
to what you consider important.
In other words, if you are not sure what is important to you,
look at what you are doing.

But now it is time to re-evaluate,
to pause and take stock,
to take another look
and see anew
what you really perceive as worthwhile.

Won't you do this, please?
Then put what is important at the helm.
Let this light your way and fuel your trip.

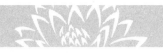

Only what is fully important can be fully compelling.
And unless you are full,
you will not experience your always-existing Fullness.

Pause again and take a look.
What are you really after?
What do you desire above all else?
Look deeply, feel deeply, sense inwardly into yourself. . .
and do not be afraid to be absolutely beautifully honest.

Desert Dance

Trees dancing in the distance like lovers reunited
leaves wisps of hair keeping tempo
moonlight glitters in silver pools of collected rain
reflecting a pale moon behind hazy clouds
electric eel snaps along the horizon
illuminating the night in red dust
quickly gone, returned to black
awaiting the growl of mother earth
as her children return to her womb
showering us with cool kisses
while earth bleeds green from brown veins
recycling her generous bounty once again

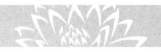

A Love Song

Your voice
Soothes honey on a cold winter day
Raspy and Rich
Fills empty space with starry nights

Your touch
Envelops me in love, healing from within
Soft and Strong
Opening locked doors without a key

This love
Eases its way past all my borders
Beckoning and Beautiful
I'm both lost and found.

Silence

Are you whispering?
Within me.

O my dearest,
there you are again!

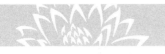
Ode to Your Loving Nature

Silky daisies, and lilies, and orchids
caressing the veil of your silvery hair,
like waterfalls from the sky—
and resting on the sweetness of your womb.
Mother Nature is waiting for your graceful foot
to touch the ground.
You open your measured dance on the whispering grass,
and squirrels and trees rejoice at the melody of your wise steps.
You are floating in space and time,
on the silent wings of a newborn butterfly,
speaking words of kindness to a restless World.
Your eyes are bathed in the fiery light of Life,
and your humane prayers are murmured to the clouds.
You're the Mother of the Sun.
You are precious.
You are Love.

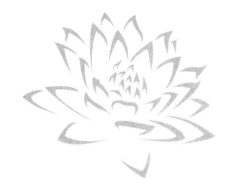

Freedom

The past is frozen
The future is melting
The present is weather

HawaH

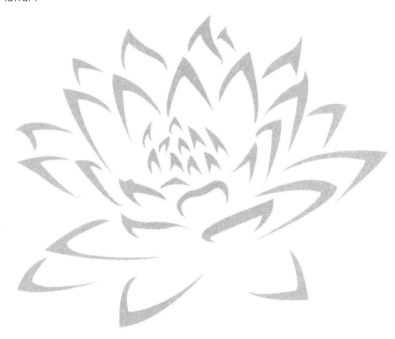

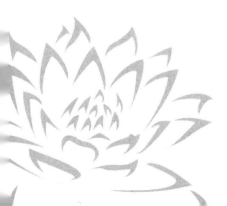

Who Am I?

A winter walk
in New England—
icy wind:
Stepping into my thoughts
I dream myself
into existence.

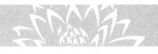

Love Cycle

Flowing from the earth,
Ever endlessly,
We are a cycle of death
And rebirth.

You are the ocean,
And I rejoice,
In joining your horizon.

The dark skies behind my eyes
Suddenly seem closer,
And shine,
Lighting up my mind.

From you I soar,
And into you I fall,
Helping you design the shores
And bedrocks,
Of our ever-changing, immortal
Existence.

Simple Request

Pointed ends of feather spines
Mark each bone and muscle of mine
I dig my teeth in scornfully, but they disregard my effort
The edges spread like drenching ink
Converging into a puzzled maze
I surrender with my palms turned in acceptance
Before the mirror
The reflection of my skin is drenched by hateful ink
Turning my white feathers to black
My eyes focus inside themselves. . .
I nod
I have been here before and I understand this quest
To shed my feathers light enough to fly
One simple form of prayer
Deep inside the privacy of my hollow chest
Socializing with the edges of pink lungs
That expand, consuming peace
This, like many other melodious moments won't last forever
Recess, respire, freeing venom from the tip
Of the snake's tongue
God help me pray more acutely
On the stones in your rivers
And the grass of your fields
Where I spun with barefooted toes and outstretched hands
The sun melting my face into submissive joy
That could not be filled or defined otherwise
Violins sing painfully
The blue befits deepness and the air is intoxicated
With intensity too rich for me to bear without crying
I groom my feathers with humble breaths of love
And leave the wicked edges outside.

Attachment

Your physical body left so quickly
I am not prepared
This was not my plan
I cannot let you leave

My inner voice asks for help in the solace of my poses
Explore the ancient ways I study and I teach

The pain does not ease
Inner God and Wise Woman do not impart guidance
I am left to sit in vast emptiness, the deepest sadness I have
ever met
The sorrow weighted
With many lifetimes and many loved ones

Time passes
Tears are less and then more
I sit now and reflect
Those fleeting moments of your physical body's death

The pain has transformed
My soul is fed by the life you divined
I am nourished
I am thankful

My heart feels broad and wide
Immense as the ocean, sky, land
I feel a light in each of my cells
I see the spread beyond physical boundaries

Our souls
And the thin veil between us

Untitled

body bends
and opens.
soft flow of ocean
floods
my heart.
once rigid
boundaries
becoming permeable.
mind witness
to the
transformation
on the mat.

Evolution

sometimes in life
there is a pain
that runs so deep
winds so tightly
about the heart
that it is no longer pain
an ache that seeps
into the core of the soul
anguish that throbs
and beats in rhythm
with the pulse
pain that burns away fear
purges past passions
and erases memory
deeper and deeper it flows
becoming part of the blood
burrowing into the bones
until it is all that remains
pain like that changes
becomes something else
develops a sort of beauty
evolves into a type of joy
consumes all else
and becomes a driving force
a reason to draw the next breath
and the next and the next
in the blind hope
that this breath
will be the one
when the pain ends

Inner Encounter

My mantras were released
they flew towards eternity
Their spell will finally break somewhere in time.

I search to be one
in another space,
another time
where love will defy
the pain of an inner distance.

My body claims this place
But my soul will escape
And that will be my last rebellion
against karma.

Words like cryptogams
come to me again
The truth lies
in front of me
while
I am no longer here.

It takes no time to realize
That this absence does not cover
any space
any measure of time
or eternity

Defiant me
here
Uncontrollable me
there

My inner encounter awaits.

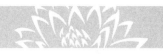

Matters

in the middle the only thing
important is
in the end
in the beginning
the only thing
in the middle the only thing really
in the middle
in the start
and in the middle the
only thing
important
is the tenderness.

nothing matters
in the end but the tenderness
the affection
in the middle

rough in the raw
in the middle
it's the affection
the indiscriminate
the case of
the ending
the love without brackets
the end of the start
and in the middle
the only
thing is the tenderness
the affection
the navel
the heart

the beginning
is always all beginning
with ending
in the middle
when you end in the middle
you begin
and begin tenderness
in the end
the only thing ending
is this

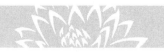

Don't Change

For my friends. We practice cooking and we
practice mind dancing. We practice practices
privately. Relationships roll across the floor.
We have as our guides train tracks alongside
highways incurvate lakesides frozen spring.
Things running next to one another.

Lapping. KING and QUEEN intersect here
and nowhere else do they curl into one another
like so many humming sections intersections
divorce. It never crossed my mind when you
touched my nipples that you left the realm of love.
Passengers on humming rails swans sleeping
ice flows. DON'T CHANGE posted everywhere
lanes change.

Words

What are words?
A half way house?
An attempt at expression?
Attempt only
Half only
Yet behind the words
The powerful stuff
Bright shining meaning
Everythingness
Nothingness
For ever and ever
Without the words
Still light and bright
Always
And so sometimes
Rest in
No words.

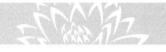

Untitled

I often sleepwalk through life
eyes open
besodden in that moment
between light and dark
hard edge and softness
springtime and summer
The Pause Between breaths
Held there, captive, hovering
Dying to be awake.

Silent Surrender

In the silence of the night,
when the inner quiet reflects the outer calm,
I converse with God.

In total surrender,
my heart breaks open.
As the last drops of Maya flow out,
joy finds room to enter.
It spreads like the dawning sunrise
creeping into every inch of a hallowed cave,
and we speak with one voice.

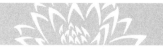

Divine Signature

love dances inside
every single atom
divine signature

One Love

Come into the light
Hold each other's hearts
Keep a tranquil mind
Full of hope and serenity
Believe anything is possible
Imagine yourself where you want to be
It will become reality

Limitless imagination will change the world
Set your intention and accomplish
Believe it and you will live it
Come together
Unite as one love

The universe is infinite unity
Universal is love
Be love
Feel love within your entire being
Let it radiate out into the world
Touch everyone you meet with your light and love

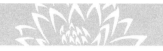

Between Words

this is not a poem of love
poems are for poets
and love
is what lives between the words

Soma from Angirasa

Sacred for its edge, soft in heart
There is nothing to achieve, less to need.
Rising with the falling breath,
whirling in the stillness of intoxication,
Soma drenches this soul and that light of heaven inside,
And you, you are that moon inside this heart.
She rises and falls in the sky, full tonight for Soma,
Full tonight as you, in me.

The Power of the Heart's Longing

I dreamt of her, lives before we met,
By seeing others that we are not,
Recognizing ourselves again, we know how
spring rain leaves leaves in wet grass,
Where hearts ache for parting and this dream a secret,
but not to her. She knows what I know.

Asanas After Troy

Anger. Tears. and a fleeting desire for violence
disrupt a dreamer's dream
of race-less love in world without lynching.

       certain moments stoke outrage-fueled flames,
       exciting anger—our sense of self's immune sytem.
       certain moments remind me that we fine folk
       are born with holes in hearts, yearning for forever.

forever seems most pleased by a reflection ever-changing
so, some ill-aim with silly ideas
that more matter alone will quench cosmic thirst.
some pillage earth, rape women, slaughter men,
kill feral folk and fauna, and disown many other beauties.

in moments like this,
       i overlook spirit's possible possession of us.
       i overlook what futures beautiful histories allude to.
         i overlook the dreamer's dream
of race-less love in world without lynching

but the ritualized returning of awareness to intention,
feeds and revives my well-aligned aim.
With this focus, i stoke the burning fire within,
sparking multiple mini-armageddons, cleansing me,
cleansing us, of enshrined criminality, foul histories, unlove,
and silly ways, becoming better within, and without.

       well postured for living the dreamer's dream
of race-less love in world without lynching.

The state of Georgia executed Troy Davis on September 21, 2011 despite serious doubts about his guilt, police intimidation of witnesses, Davis's steadfast profession of innocence, and a complete lack of physical evidence.

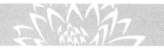

Notes Throughout a Day

::7:42am::
morning stillness makes space for sweet songs
morning movement lends grace to the mixings
of magic and muscle
morning presence massages soils
planted with love seeds,
and nursed wth sweet toils.

::11:37am::
at the meeting
of pockets of eternity
and the beauties of biology,
i find a tender reverence.

::2:10pm::
i soak in sun
and awaken muscle
i dig roots deep down
into the rockbed of love
and i bloom beauty and laughter
echoing hereafter. . .

::11:07pm::
i let go and whisper sparkle black incantations
transfixing through tough tongue spells
and deep drinks in god's great well.
i coax dreams of an ancient love, and mistle-toed teeth.
dreams of spirit animals and peanut butter.
dreams of soon-to-be us-histories aware of the unseen.
i let go to the free frolics in eyelid land,
swirling in the redness of closed-eye sight. . .

::3:42am::
a cosmonaut of consciousness,
i am buoyed by energies both below and above,
a fine vessel i float on warm lakes of love.

This Burden

I did not ask for this burden
when one becomes two
In a moment
everything changes
that is when a teacher is needed

—chop wood carry water—

this is only the beginning
As the old Shaman will tell his
apprentice
"I am sorry that you have become
enlightened,
Now get back to work"

Waking up is nothing
living free and undetected
in a world without vision
that is the challenge

How do you speak a language
that has no words?

Letter from a Secret Admirer

Don't torment yourself with uncertainty—
I hear your every word to me,
your every frustration,
your every impassioned cry
for a way out of your confusion.
I watch you forgive
the same people
again and again.
And you ask for my forgiveness, too,
for what you call, "turning your back on me."
But I assure you, my precious,
no forgiveness is necessary.
All those years you lashed out at the world,
I kept watch over you,
never stopped loving you,
never stopped rooting for you.
It's not easy seeing someone suffer so.
It takes as much courage and faith
as the one who chose to suffer.
For you see, my child, this is what you asked for,
and I granted, because I, too, wanted to see you grow.
I—even more than you—
wanted to see you transcend your cherished fallacy
that life is a tragedy.
I—even more than you—
wanted to see you triumph
over the challenges you face.
Please don't doubt that I hear your prayers.
In my silence
is my undying desire
for you to hold out your hand
and invite me to dance.
For you see, my love, I—even more than you—
long for *your* embrace.

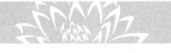

Melting into the One

we are all melting into one another
like a popsicle in the Sun—
it is messy
it is fragrant and full of color—
enjoy it as a Child would!
do not grab a napkin
or clean
do not worry about the result
but be in the moment
tasting the fruits of Life

The Mystics Drink Tea

The mystics were never mystics.
They were so very practical
And also difficult.

Who wants to be bothered with worldly things.
Not I.
I want to drink the nectar of God

And here on Earth this tea.
It is a ceremony and a dialogue
Even for the mystic who does not speak

Much at all. With the taste of it
Divine Mother fills the throat
And there is much to be said

of what is important. Often people
speak of nothing. This is fine.
People should speak more often

of the unfurling flower. Look into your
lover's eye and you will see it.

The Lovers' Manifesto

we are lovers and dreamers because we become like water
in the constant pursuit of moving and shaking
what the universe has bestowed upon us in its perfect
diction of Saturday afternoon picnics.

we refuse to stagnate, withdraw, give-up, escape
for more than a few hours at a time.
we see life for the process and have always loved
happiness for its sexy elusiveness.
in turn, we have learned to love
her twin sister of heartbreak
and how it comes to leave us a different person,
knowing more about beauty and kindness
than we thought possible.

we believe in:
dancing as prayer, chewing slowly, asking questions
and listening to the answers, impromptu morning mass
on deserted mountain tops, delirious gratitude,
homemade bread, riveting conversation,
and cups of tea when the moment requires rest.

we are not afraid of change,
our bodies, getting older, technology, confusion,
bursts of anger, or the elusiveness of everything we seek.
we have learned to sit still
to see that which reaches beyond us
and connects every single part of this world.
by seeing the connection,
we finally know there is no more need to fight.

we are fed by each other, lessons learned,
childrens' sticky faces, treetops waving in the breeze,
and above all, the love that loves to love us.
we tough it out, we change, and we will change
this world through consideration,
compost piles of ideas,
and a willingness to laugh in the face of anything
that seems too big, too closed, or too difficult.
we make loving look good.

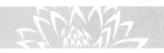

Moments

There have been a hundred thousand moments
since we last spoke.

Across the world,
each moment has contained a million memories.

Each one,
for me,
has contained a thought of you.

Seeking You

Is my heart crying out in pain
or softly singing your name?

Are my fingers stiff and slick
with unwelcome cold and rain
or wetted by drops of your grace?

Is my intrusive loneliness
and craving for human comfort
demanding that I board
the busload of crowded bodies

or whispering a secret

I can find you deeply
deeply hidden
within the cave
of my own heart.

My face, reflected
in the mirror of time
insults me with the indelicacy of aging

Will I be able to outrun
the racing hours and days
to fall into your arms
before the flesh crumbles
and I am thrown onto the wheel
of revolving lifetimes?

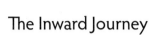

The Inward Journey

Walking the mandala of the mind,
the inward spiral, the shadowed depths,
each step closer to the darkness's center
is a step closer to the lightened edge.

Dermatographica

I can draw with dry fingernails
lines on my skin, red welts that rise up on my forearms
my skin remembers touch by the way it chafes
I can trace dry fingernails over goosebumps on my calves
and tell stories about this sick superpower
and its beautiful Latin name
dermatographica
skin writing
I have spent afternoons drawing names beneath itchy sweaters
when I remember I add details
cities
favourite books
profiles looking out of windows,
unmade beds

I have been carving out pounds of sacred flesh,
each marked with a name
and a portrait in perfect inflammation
I have been wrapping them in packages
then placing them in mailboxes
next to empty milk bottles and flyers for takeout Chinese

I have wondered if they were opened like gifts
if these lonely dermal stories were left out on kitchen counters,
framed in bedrooms, cooked and eaten.
I have wondered if these bits of flesh reminded them of me.

I was asked to perform this feat once, by two doctors,
men, they crossed their arms, laughed, glanced at each other

I want to believe they felt awe
I want to believe they would have liked to have seen
their own names
"Dr." neatly dotted on the hip crest
before the name along the thigh

I carved them out pieces, small gifts, a line of hamstring
and one tensor fascia latae
but I didn't remember their names.
I wrote "Doctor" on both packages, wrapped them carefully,
left them side by side on the examination table.

I have given these pounds of flesh freely
these perfect gifts, each branded and sent away

Because I wanted to see my ribcage,
the delicate curve of my collarbone
I've wanted to see the ridges of my spinal column
the apertures of my sacrum
tendons peeling away from my kneecap
like a careful hand
I've always wondered if my bones have scars
if they have writing on them
I've wanted to know whose name was etched
on my skeleton
beneath all the moveable flesh
I have hoped
it was mine

Adina's Soul (Where Revolutionaries Come From)

I carried this poem in a place so deep
That
40 weeks later
It had its own heartbeat
Our chatty talks
Transformed innocently
Into chemistry
Sugarcane so sweet
That 72 hours later
Tantric tears called for
Veins and bloodstreams
A rotating blood clot
Fueled by blissful
Wistful pelvic raindrops
I carried this poem in a place so deep
That
Our innocent
Synergistic
Overtly casual
Covertly sensual encounters became so sugarcane sweet
That moonlit shadows pouncing off window panes
Left meticulous stains
That glistened and crystallized into a whole new being
I carried this poem in a place so deep that
Your wet became my dry
And my hot became your cold
And ten months later our revolutionary, cabbalistic synergy
Became our
I
And Adina's soul
Became our reason
WHY.

She Walks in Two Worlds

She walks in two worlds
That become one
At the zipper toothed seam
Where her toes meet the earth
The soles of her feet
Thumping out the beat
Of drums that have been pounding
Steady like her heart
For millennia
Her hips sway in time with the ocean tides
Constantly bringing to shore
The sea foam of her desire
Playing cradle to her abdomen
Filled with hope
For love and the eternity
Of creation
Her deepest longing
To be the zero point of life
The nest out of which fly
A thousand generations of untethered souls
All calling her
Mother
Matriarch
Ancestor
Myth
Her chest blooms with milky white lilies
Blossoming out in Fibonacci sequences
From the blush pink center
Providing nectar
For bees and butterflies
Lovers and hummingbirds
Seeking sweet nourishment

From the heart
Her neck and shoulders
Create a soft landing place
For weary heads
Concentrating the scent
Of amber and rose
That transmutes her soul
Into a sweet smelling offering
To the Gods
Lips that hold secrets
Too big and beautiful
For the world to handle
Right now
Speak bold pronouncements
Of the explosion to come
Her hair
Thick, flowing waves
Of intricately spun gold
Thinly veil her crown
A lotus blossom
Spiraling out into the unknown known
She walks in two worlds
That become one
At the infinitesimally small point
Where her head meets the sky

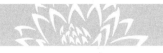

Untitled

There is something inside me
That sees you
And remembers
A lifetime
When you were my brother
My father
My lover
My friend
And I wonder
What I forgot in that lifetime
That you are here to teach me again
And I wonder
What I forgot in that lifetime
That needs to be remembered
So I look again
And I search your eyes
For the answer
Because maybe that answer
Is the key to it all
The lesson I need
To reach nirvana
The roadmap to heaven
I wait
I wonder
I hope you will reveal it soon
So that I can memorize
Every moment
And hold the secret in my heart
Until the next lifetime
When the me that is me
Will see the you that is you
And I will pray to the stars
To let me forget again

The Elevator

the door that
almost closed
was opened.

will the door
that did close
open again?

Evocation

in the abyss
of the lack of
understanding
that often
masquerades
as truth,
may we the
evolving,
living
among we the
dead and dying,
mesmerized
by the illusion of
power and control &
blind acceptance of
value systems
birthing our current
state of bondage
recall!
may we the
pre-conscious
bond
with we the
un-conscious
in this the
age of
grace and
In-light-enment
remembering
who we were
and who we
in fact, still are.

Shakti Breath

I return to the mat
a place of refuge.
My body an altar,
an offering to Shakti.
Some days I struggle to do the warm-ups.
I avoid all the slim bodies on the cover
of the yoga books and tapes,
the ones that are twisted up like pretzels,
their smile exudes peace and joy.
As if they came into this world like clay—moldable
with ease of movement—swan-like grace.
I am frustrated by the measuring stick inside my head and
their looks that say I must spend lifetimes trying to
puzzle out
the keys to health and happiness.
Why is my karma different?
I wear my weight like a neon sign
yet, I feel pulled to connect to my breath—
that column of eternal light that Shakti rides
up and down my spine seeking her mate at my crown.
I can't always touch my own inner beauty,
or my toes,
but if I stay with my breath
my body loosens just enough
to go a little further than I did yesterday.

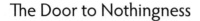

The Door to Nothingness

No one can do this work for you.

The work of Breathing.

The work of Letting Go.

No one can take away your Self for you—
That heavy Self of infinite burden.
No one can do this work for you.
The work of Silence.

Only you can open this
Singular Door to Nothingness
Where stark colorless pervasive wind blows,
Where there exists only One Solitary Knowing.
And in that paradoxically unconfined room
Of One Choice—One Choice Alone—
There is, curiously enough,
freedom

Singing,
Silent,
Totally silent,
No choice,
One total omnipresent choice,

come home.

The Yoga Teacher

The time is now.
It has always been now, but now
It is now more than ever.
I do not know you.

The silence that sits between us
Is very thick and full
As if it's more real than any utterance
We sort of make, like
Two really old people
Or two quite young people,
One or the other,
But we're not adults here, we're
Lost aged masters or
Clumsy foolish adolescents.

I do not know you.
I do not know your story.
I do not know the channels
Your mind and heart swim.
But I watch you move
I sense you being
I hear you speak.

I am old, I am young
I know too much, I don't know anything
I've got a hundred stories, I've got none
And maybe you're just another one—
Another one of those hundred stories—
Those flames that swear to fade with time.

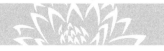

Hope seems like a lost cause
Hope seems like gambling in Vegas
But I've never been to Vegas
Let's drive there
Take a road trip together
We'll take the silence with us
That rich full thick silence
It'll keep us company
While we forget who we ever thought we were
While we dig into each other's fires
Listening for that sudden yet
Anticipated
Moment
When
Everything
Drops

Transcendence

Transcendence is an apocalyptic event
It takes the past as it leaves the present
Change is always the same
If you care to look deeper into it
It is form passing into form
It is orgasmic
It is the expansion of truth and reality
Through the phases of duality
Like the moon it moves from necessity
Guaranteed full promised monthly
This is bold like love is bold
Naked revealed
It has no body and nobody can have it
Love that is...has no body
and no body has love
Love is the body
Blood, the intoxication the invitation
To this apocalypse
This standing naked
Psyche stripped is the flesh
The matter is the mind
Thought is form
Words come next
Few make new most make do.

Shut Up and Listen

Only these few words to describe all of this
Hardly does it seem fair
More likely it appears arrogant for one person
To speak so many millions of words in a lifetime
Saying this or that about this and that
It hardly seems fair
To say anything
To describe what can be seen with even the
Most enchanting schemes of words
Is barely enough
And yet
We think we have seen it all and can tell it
Like it is or was
But all we are doing is showing a small corner
Of a shadow of it and even that is a lie
Truth is immense
It is larger than the universe
Words wiggle out of minds filled with images
Linked together as a sequence of events in time
We cannot know what we are talking about
Until we are willing to stop talking
And break out of our small corner to reach
For possibilities that cannot be described
How to do that is to enter the mystical land of
Shut up and listen

The Silence of Us All

There are 7 billion human beings on the planet they say
Each one going about their business
While 150 million land animals are put to death every day
Making 56 billion a year can you spin it?
6 million dead every hour
100,000 die in a minute
27 billion slaughtered each year
Just in our Land of the Free - Home of the Brave
As we go about the important business of the day

Why should we bother?
Animals are animals you might say
They eat each other every day

No Way!......wait!
The animals who we eat, the cows, goats, and sheep,
Are vegetarians who do not eat meat
Unless it is forced down their throats
Which is quite an easy feat
These creatures are docile by nature
But we human beings
Trying our best to make a buck
We don't even give a flying _____
After all it is only some poor slob
Chained in a stall who cannot speak after all

Besides isn't that what God put them here for?

If we want to reduce the fear in our own lives
In our country, city, town, neighborhood, home
In our nervous systems, then why not start with something
Near by, close to home
Most of us interact with animals three times a day
When we sit down to eat them

Instead of exploiting all the mothers
Couldn't we try to improve this relationship?
Who give milk, eggs and birth to babies
Only to live lives of mourning.

Babies taken from their mothers
Mother dripping tears and milk
While we capitalize on their loss
And harvest the white liquid from the nipple
As we dribble and talk "conversation"
Meeting in restaurants and cafes
When are we going to be kind
How many rhymes will it take
To cause us to pause before we order that
Burger and Shake?

Speak out.
What better way?
If you won't speak,
What are you busy saying?
Whatever else you had to say,
It's not worth that much today.

Beyond the Pentagon: Dreaming of Allen Ginsberg, 1970

O Ganga-mouthed Ginsberg,
you lit Varanasi incense.
We sat on Whitman's leaves.
The sun revealed the
seven gates of green.

Doves flapped
inside your heart,
flew out of your Om,
soared on the current
of your gold-threaded breath.

A poem filled the sky,
our eyes collided.
We prayed to the fallen
not for grace,
but for now.

A tiger crouched
then roared.
The earth opened
like your woman hole
and took us wholly home.

Surya Namaskar

Biking to work this late—May morning
I feel the drizzle through my jean jacket
and sweatshirt. Not a drenching but a mist
on the skin, long and slow, just what the lawn
needs for the new grass I planted. Today I teach

Surya Namaskar hoping to bribe the hiding sun
with attention. So much rain. I have a student
who is dying. She joins us if she can after chemo
or radiation. Today, as she lay down, she cried.
She doesn't know if she has a week, three months

or years. One by one, her windows are closing.
One eye no longer focuses. She's nauseous
from the Tamoxifen. While the rest of us stand,
she sits in a chair and moves her arms. Inhale,
I instruct, let your arms stretch outward

from your heart. Exhale, palms together, gather
the universe back within. Inhale, arms reach
for the sun. Exhale, bend down and touch the earth.
"While I'm in class doing yoga," she says,
"I know that everything is right with the world."

The Shape My Bones Are In

My kneecaps would make
great earmuffs for the
hear-no-evil monkey.

Squirrels want to curl
in my soft-sculpture hip sockets
and hibernate till spring.

Is it my sacrum or a flounder,
seduced by the worm on my tailbone?
Don't get hooked, I warn, unheeded.

The heart and lungs dangle
like fruit bat trapeze artists
in the net of my rib cage.

Only a hole in the center
of my skull, my rhinoceros nose
knows physics and won't apologize.

When I die, don't cremate me, please.
Let the snake hoist me up
by my stirrup sitting bones

so I can fold flat
like an ironing board
and slack-clack-rattle in the breeze.

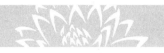

Oh, Pilgrim Heart

You travel to and from source
bringing with you from the womb
treasures and secrets
that are only received in whispers
from the Divine.

The journey in is paved with
those familiar landmarks;
Patterns and habits
dot the deserted landsacpe
like mirages in the distance. . .
beckoning.

Moments feel suffocating.

. . .This too shall pass. . .

Lying at the feet of the Mother
worn and weary from the relentless journey
in and up.
Rest here, for a while my beloved.

In Her bosom of Infinite Peace
and Love.

Bask in the warm glow,
steady gaze
of the Divine.

Gathering up every speck of
wisdom and light you can hold,
a balancing 8 limbed act,
you hold fast to the fullness.

Trusting the strength of the
cord umbilical to life
that binds you to the Self.

Like an experienced mountaineer,
carrying with you Supreme Love and Infinite Wisdom;
you leave the cave of the heart to root your being back
into the world.

You seek out suffering and pain
and selflessly bestow the gifts of unconditional
love and light you so carefully hold
at the core of your being.

Oh Pilgrim Heart!

May your countless journeys
on this river of light
bless you with grace and discernment
to see the Supreme Self in every wanderer you meet.

Hold most tight—
the cord that binds you to your own light,
and remember this is the most noble journey
you shall ever take.

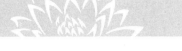

Wake Up, Wake Up

Days begin and end
arising intention, saluting the sun,
only an hour to get done.

Reverence to cycle:
Heartbeats to become, come to be, hearts beat as one.

Yielding, folding into:
Separation from dissensions, tensions to be loved.

Unfolding into the behind us,
engaged, it can be done.
Breath, attention, flooding into life,
Letting go, distensions, letting go to write...

Inhale, prana to wake the might
mind gone plank, chatter rung, exhaling,
to a quieted height.
"Down dog!"
Heels, relaxing down,
to the earth,
mind-full pleas
wander less to adventure,
pleased minds filled with wonder,
of breath, of beauty, of light.

Building heat, fire, opening:
A sauna in each body, teacher's delight.

Tried, untired, true, we trust, aligning right...

Warmth filled, radiating bodily lights
a class, together of believers, in sync, flexible,
balanced in sight.

The "I can" becomes the "I did," to the perpetuating "I am,"
harmonize with the feat of receivers
of those who understand.

One body, one light, one life to be within
each moment, choosing our mats,
letting our daze go, gaze within.
Finding inner truth, a side, no separation in this vessel.

Water filled, clean, flowing, the benefit to nourish, to care, to be:
The love of today from within
the love of the infinite one,
The love in we.

We Are Fish

We are fish swimming
in a sea of majesty,
asking everyone we meet
for a drink that will quench
our fierce fire of longing.

Perhaps it is this that enables us
to grow wings, so that we may leave
the ocean, however briefly,
and obtain a glimpse of the
somewhere else we long to be.

We fall back, only to rise again,
over and over
convinced that our flight
is liberating us
from our longing.

What trickery.
The ecstatic state
of seeing the great expanse of sky
leaves us gasping for the water
we have just left.
We must leave water for air to realize
that all along we were swimming
in the majesty of our longing.

The trickery goes farther,
for in the end we realize that all along
we have been our majesty
swimming in Itself.

Transformation

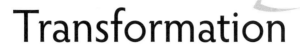

There is nothing more I want
Than to join you in the cocoon

To know the dreams
That grow wings

Butterfly,
What is your
Dream?

HawaH

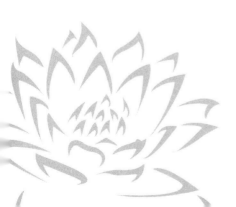

The Practice

A moment in God's wilderness
Confirmed what eagles knew,
That we, like ants to minds of boys,
Are granted purpose in the ploys,
Yet filled with lust for transient toys,
Have long forgotten why we do.

An hour upon God's ocean sand
Sets slow the orb of gold.
Wondrous, yet my mortal mind
Gropes within to reason find—
My impermanence to Nature bind—
Remake my crumbling ego bold.

But wakeful, watchful tender Spirit
Smiling shuns the moment's tread.
The breath of 50 years sighs,
Softly, soon my heart replies,
Weaving threads of life it cries,
"Be wakeful soon for you'll be dead."

The urgent plea from deep within
Makes me wonder where I've been.
Must coming years repeat the sin,
The great illusion that I win.

I bow down low, take off my hat,
Step humbly on my yoga mat.

Gift

35 ridiculously capable carpenters
a foreman who was mercifully absent
(doubtless chasing skirts in town)
two top-notch operations consultants
a mergers and acquisitions team from
the city of Brotherly Love
and 13 black sea turtles
(who are not by the way black)

were assembled recently in my head.
They worked without fail for
One hundred and eight nights.

They built a platform there
Of the finest love titanium
It is perfectly balanced
leveled with a brand new compassion gauge
Cabled with humility steel

It is a safe place from which
You can teach me.
There is nothing in this world you can do wrong
As my beloved teacher.

This platform surrounds you
With reverence, respect, and appreciation.
Teach me.

Hamstrung

Practicing forever.
Trying harder than
an ant
moving a fallen tree
alone, on his back
without straps.

My crazy head is still
Thirty feet away
from my laughing feet.

Outside the studio
A gibbous moon rises
Fat in the sky
Soon, like me, to die

There is no choice but to let go
no choice, but let go
Let choice go.

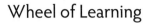

Wheel of Learning

Can I tell you "bow your head"
failing to bow silently, alone on my mat?
I dig, I listen, I mine.
Not to be great as a teacher.
I dig to save myself
from the enormous sadness
of faking it.
Because Yoga is a "lifestyle choice"
like the Dalai Lama is a monk.
Svadhyaya is optional
like holding your breath underwater.
The teaching is as deep as the teacher.
so pray that your limbs remain attached:
pray until your arms fall off.

Hey Divine Force!

I want to fall
Deeply enough
in love with
you in me

That I see you
wrapped in others
and love them

such that
molecules and atoms
In their hearts

Spontaneously
Regenerate
Love.

I have no idea how to
Pull this one off.
Could you hook me up with that?

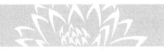

All Connected

This bone-joint-ligament-muscle-fatty-liquid frame
sack of shit and piss

All of this soon ends in stink and dust
what's the value of greed and lust?

A wood house in the wind
twigs, branches, boards and splinters
water washing through the city
it's heart pulsing the blood of the people

Movement as natural as
sushumna rising
magnetized
solar and lunar poles
spine supple strong steady

A channel aligned
out from the body
rests the power of the mind
awaiting commands
translating vibrations into thought
seeking it's solace/center

Source
the quietude of the soul
somewhere between nothing and everything
a momentary pause
in the spinning of the wheel

Metaphysical Property

Location, location, location

Real estate—boom!

There's almost not enough room for me to see the sky
so I salute to the sun inside

Reaching up and back bending low lunging pyramiding

Myself strong
foundation feet planted
I shall not be moved.

Parivrtta

As the nights grow cold
I fold inward
Examine
Where are the brittle places
That can wither
And fall away like leaves?
A poem or a prayer,
The turning of the heart.
Let me find
The darknesses and angers
I no longer need
Kiss them
like old friends
And send them away into morning,
Watch them
As they twist to the light
Like sunflowers.

A Wish

to be vibrant, to be healthy. to speak when the moment
strikes. to look forward. to not pause or hesitate or be lost
in translation or forgotten in a stale cloud of mediocrity. to
accept without resignation. to move beyond the anxiety of
doubt or disbelief or lack of faith. to get good sleep. to stretch
and breathe. . .inhale. . .exhale. . .giving thanks for this moment
and these bodies.

to start this day with loving grace, bless us all and kiss your
face. to dance naked in the firelight with a full moon high in
the sky shining bright. to love with all that i have, and when
it's difficult and needed, more. to lie next to you, beside you,
inside of you.

to play. to spin lights and sticks and dance and do simple
yet beautiful tricks. to perform, for me and you. . .. . .i might even
show up wearing neon colored clown shoes. to hear the
music, even when it stops. to feel the rush of waves. to
actively create the connections and ways that will sustain us
as we experience darker days,—so roll with it.

to be vibrant, healthy. to put one sure foot in front of the other,
taking me to where i'm going and arriving with each step.
to dream wide awake, imagining the possibilities while
planting flowers in the desert.

to ask. to remember. forget. hold on and let go. to circle the
ancient tower and shapeshift.

if i had just one, that'd be my wish.

Hatha

At dawn the sun sits on the horizon
emerging from the Gulf
solid and brazen
fire drenched red,
while the moon slumbers
full and pale in the morning sky.
I stand on the beach
warm from the bed
strung between the vision of two forces:
pulled by the coolness of the moon,
intrigued by the flames of the sun:
like a pendulum
delicately balanced in the hazy light.
My eyes drawn,
my mind,
dazed
needing the moon's cool clarity.

HA - THA -
sun moon,
light dark,
life death
ultimate perfect union,
dancing in the earth's vibration.
Orbiting around our planet
constant and firm,
pre-historic
witnesses
as we clamor
for more and more

now, today,
as we daily plunge,
with consistent abandon,
into ultimate destruction.

HA THA
sun moon
rising setting
eclipsing
melding one into the other
perfect union.

I stand between the two
and try to feel
the essence
of perfect symmetry
right between the eyes:
heart of fire
quiet mind
one body
one soul
setting
rising
now
and
only
now.

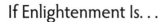

If Enlightenment Is. . .

If enlightenment is a destination,
then I don't want to go there.
If life is suffering
and nothing else,
then the Buddha can keep it.
If Heaven is a fluffy vacation,
then cancel my ticket.
If sainthood is obedience
and nothing else,
then no halo will ever fit me.
If Jesus never laughed,
then he is not my savior.
If goddessence is male
and nothing else,
then call me a disbeliever.

But if She swings,
and has a sense of humor,
if her prophets
brew a bit of mischief
on the rough side of town,
if life is a mystery
and enlightenment
can be found and lost
any where?

Then let's play this game!
Let's jump that train!
Let's cry and laugh,
suffer and indulge,
fall and bounce,
dance in the cremation ground.
Let's play a drinking game
called duality
and fight sometimes,
often, just
for the Hell of it.
If Heaven is not a place
then you will find me there
lost in the throes of desire
and fulfillment
strutting and fretting
my hour upon the stage
acting out a tale
full of silence and bliss
signifying everything.

Pain Suite

Pain is a flower
most folks pull from their garden
thinking it common.

How precious and rare
to be born in a human body
even angels lust.

Some say that Yoga
is soft. Easy. For wimps. Yes.
No. It is a mirror.

Miracles do not blossom
In the intense heat
Of skepticism.

Some pain is torture.
Some, pleasure. The difference?
How I ask for it.

A rose with no thorns
Is a teacher with no truth
A bowl with no food.

Inside every rock
A silent Buddha waiting
For the stone carver.

Grandma's Ghost

Grandma's ghost spoke
through the lips of a shaman:
"I never wished this life for you!"
Grandma was a superstitious woman
who communed with spirits
and studied Egyptian mysticism.
She was as careful
to keep us kids away
from her astrology books
as the bottle of whiskey
she kept in her sock drawer.
"This Life" of interaction
with the unseen and drunken
one foot in both worlds
and now her also
using the medium
she asked me to avoid.
What am I up to,
that she would return
sixteen years later
with a warning?
I teach Yoga to seven-year-olds
and stressed-out CEO's.
How many evil spirits
am I likely to encounter
in a million-dollar fitness center?
Legions, it turns out.
We all walk with an invisible posse
Of ancestors, angels and demons,
legacy of an American lifestyle
fueled by petroleum imperialism.
Even homeless bums
sleep on illegal concrete.

San Francisco was stolen from the Mexicans,
who stole it from the Ohlone Indians,
who stole it from the pelicans.
At least the natives prayed
to the animals they ate.
When I read a statistic
that less than one percent
of the world is wealthy enough
to keep loose change by the bed,
it put into perspective
the privilege of teaching kids yoga
at ten dollars a head.
This is no sermon on morality or righteousness,
this is a meditation on what IS.
Good and Evil
are everyone's neighbors.
The path to enlightenment
meanders from rose garden
to the rough side of reality
disturbingly often.
"This life" means a lot of grave digging. . .
my own.
"Self-Discovery" includes the buried bones of past karmas,
the inherited debt of one's ancestors:
White Privilege, Alcoholism, Incest.
It is difficult to find
an empty plot in this cemetery,
earth soaked in blood, hip deep in mud,
my shovel striking hard truths
and strangely shaped memories.

To most folks, Ego death
looks a lot like regular death.
In India, they say
an American birth
is an opportunity
to cash in on good karma
and enjoy an easy life on Earth.
Here I am, spending my vacation
as an amateur archeologist,
sorting gold teeth and wedding rings.
Identifying every body
as another aspect of Self:
Blissfully Ignorant Imperialist
Me again.
Racist In Recovery
Me again
Whiteboy mystic.
Me again.
A cosmos unfolding
Me again.
Grandma, thanks for your warning
but don't bother mourning,
Charles is already dead.
Ekabhumi cleaning up his mess.
Heaping mantras on the heart's fire
like logs on Chuck's funeral pyre.
Planting flowers in the family plot.
He left behind no ghost
Only flames like petals
Of the reddest rose.

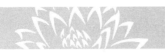

Attention

How many cups of tea
Have I wasted and let grown cold.

How many breaths
Have passed unwatched.

Spaces Between Words

the curse of friendliness
i can't find a spot
to stand in silence

hallas! enough!
i need to find
the spaces between the words
the words between the sentences
the sentences between the paragraphs
the paragraphs that build the chapters
of this new story
being born in my blood

there is a fire inside
burning through
at the fingertips
waiting to be painted
with words streaked red
like an angry sunset
spreading across
a pearl-grey sky

i like it better
when the wind whispers love songs
tickling my waiting, willing ear
the mountain offers up
ancient scents
and mysteries
histories
unwritten
unspoken
unknown

echoed within
blood and bone

all falls short
so I surrender to this madness
and
dance for Krishna with Mirabai
cry for Shamz with Rumi
seek the Bridegroom with St. John of the Cross
succumb to the agony of love with Beloved Teresa

I look
behind your face
falling into
the light
that shines through everything.

In the Unknown

This is an adventure
and there are always risks
no one is unchanged
by love
just as
no one is unchanged
by war
birth
death

creation and destruction
walk hand in hand
faith
and doubt
are the same breath

the seed
does not become the tree
without first breaking the shell
that contains the seed

the new sprout
tender and white
not even green yet
no sun to strengthen its fight for growth

yet it reaches
trusting in the light
as yet unknown
that dwells beyond the dark of the womb

and so we quest
reaching beyond the edges
breaking through the hard shell
a chick breaking through her egg

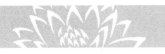

birth
is never an easy transition
not for mother
nor child
yet
the time comes
and there is no way to hold back

we
break through the gate
water flooding
the edges
erasing the ages
wearing slowly
upon the rock

trace the threads of time;
every canyon
was once a plane
then a stream
then a river
than a gorge
than a chasm
water
and wind
wearing even stone
to sand

who are we
to think
we can withstand?

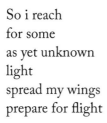

So i reach
for some
as yet unknown
light
spread my wings
prepare for flight

cell by cell
i shed my skin
in this revelation
new life begins
a kid in milk
a tree at seedling
i reach for the light

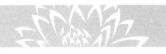

Love in the Ocean

I made love to the ocean today. . .
Wrapped my legs around her waves
Dug my fingers into her sandy back

I made love to the ocean. . .
Dove head first into bubbles foaming at her mouth
My hair was pulled out of its braids
By her salty determined waters

Actually, I might be mistaken
Maybe it was the ocean that made love to me?

She wrapped her kelp around my wrists
Squeezed me into one of her shells

I think I made the hermit crabs jealous. . .
and the dogs bark at her

For a minute I wondered what would happen
If we married and had children?

Would the dolphins finally move out of the house. . .
and the jellyfish grow brains?

I made love today,
but it's probably nothing like those
with them dirty minds think

You see, I didn't use any protection
stripped down naked
and dove right in.

Offering

I had no incense to offer you...

My hands were empty
I had no tidings
My shoes were worn and muddy
I knew not what you would expect of me
I made some wrong decisions.

I came and walked around your temple
Doing rounds of 108
I lost count halfway in between
I knew not if I should return to the beginning and count again
I knew not what I should say when I was before you
The rain had me damp
From the burden of a tumultuous journey.

Searching
Always seemingly searching
For what I could possibly offer...

Religion was obscure
But, not wanting to miss any opportunity to know you
I surrendered to every holy place and faith I came across.

I came seeking direction
Walked circles around your statues
I knew not what to offer
My hands were empty
The fruit I had not purchased
From the woman selling alms outside your gate.

I entered nonetheless
Hungry and thwarted by a self-imposed loneliness
And, I was unsure if I was to feed you. . .
Or, you were to feed me?

At times, I even felt unsure of how to pray.

I came as a wanderer
Wanting to offer something
Yet not knowing what
Finally, I decided
I would offer myself.

Savasana

Sweetheart
She whispered softly in my ear.
Wake up.
I brush away the words,
willing them to be carried past me on a breeze.
It is time
Again the whisper I try to ignore.
Surrender
I try to will away the sounds of bustling, shuffling, scattering,
awakening that surrounds me.
I lay,
In peace,
In one piece,
In the only perfect moment of stillness I own.
And still she whispers
Open your eyes.
Go away!
Re-engage.
Please don't make me!
Her voice is my own and draws circles of comfort
on my soul like caresses
Come on love, I am love, you are love,
there will be stillness again
Tomorrow.

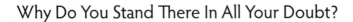

Why Do You Stand There In All Your Doubt?

why do you stand there in all of your doubt?

don't you know that your whole life has led you
to this moment. . .preparing you?

your feet have grown rooted and firm. . .
the result of all those storms you weathered.
yours are the feet that stand their ground.

your legs are powerful. . .
a strength built from trudging
through some rough and dangerous terrain.
yours are the legs that move mountains.

your shoulders are broad. . .
as they are practiced in carrying
not only the load you have been given,
but often bearing the bundle of another.
yours are the shoulders that hold others up.

all the tears you shed have cleared your vision. . .
giving you a greater capacity to see all that is there—
and who are there
before you.

yours are the eyes that not only look into the eyes of another
but the heart of another as well.

and your heart, my friend, has only grown bigger. . .
each time it was broken and patched back together.
yours is the heart that no longer
knows limits in its capacity to love.

even your hands are not the hands you began with. . .
for now their grasp is tighter and their grip is stronger.
yours are the hands of understanding.

i know you are shaking.
its true—the challenge that lies before you
is like none you've faced before.

i know you are tired.
and you should be.
you've struggled long and hard to get
where you stand now.

but i promise you, all that you've ever endured or enjoyed,
relished in or suffered with, each time you won—
but even more the times you didn't. . .
have all played their part in escorting you to this place.

your edge.

and it's not the place you stop.

oh no.
it's the place from which you'll begin.

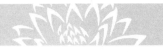

Transformations

The green transfusion of
Light growing out of your iris
Is a vine of diplomacy
Curving up towards me down
District solstice beats
Caked in trees and dirt bare
On my feet
Your hands fluctuate under laughter
Spirit calls and djembe beats
My ribcage to a moonbeam breathless
We look through willow walls and damp heat
Vine wrapped in vine
Light transfusions meet

And it's the first for me
To grow into the arms of this willow tree
Atop the stillness
Behind frozen sound
Waving over
You are
Chrysanthemum and honeydew
Wrapped in smiles
Of this fractal moment
Where we see
We are nothing more
Than green dust transfusions
Light
And sun beats

Savvy and Soulful

I drink mochas and I meditate
I wear Nikes but never eat meat
I do yoga, tai chi and I visualize
I facebook, I blog and I tweet

Occasionally I pour a martini
Daily I sip on green tea
I reflect in contemplation
on how I came to be

My laptop, ipod and cell phone
suit my savvy inclinations
my chakras align to enjoy
the kindest of soulful sensations

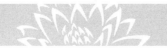

"You" Inspire God

If the hands of a clock
The shifting of digital dots
Would pull us all together
The world would be
One giant
Thundering heart
In the purest mind
Seeing with the clarity of
Timelessness

What Dedication Did I Make Again?

Thoughts have slipped through me
through cracks in the floor,
through vertebrae tingling
joints loose, hips liberated

I lay under cover, sand bag grounding me
lavender floating in the air
makes its way through my nostrils
ujjayi ceased, shallow breathing

I am thinking about my errands for the week
I am worrying about how to resolve a problem
when I get home
I am calculating bills
I am aware of a car sloshing through the puddles outside

I am interrupted by a person's untimely cough
I am pondering my regrets
I am melancholy remembering my departed friend
I am planning which tea to drink after my practice

Still I lay still
I am perfectly warm and cool
Equilibrium
"Find your drishti"

I lay feeling my lower back
and measure it's ache and release
my pelvis is grateful for the attention
"Moola bandha, baby!"

My feet are relieved
to be done with their job
of holding me up
in veera and warrior poses

Shoulders and neck aching
from the dogs carried up and down
mountains erected,
trees stretched towards the sky
Greetings to the sun
legs proving their magic by holding me up
to stand with eagles then to sit with pigeons
Breathe and melt through it

Next time I will open into wheel
just
a little
longer

What was my dedication again?

And just as I am letting my thoughts flow
through the creases of my mind
Acharya rings a gentle bell
three times it resonates louder

It tugs me into reality
I stretch, reach and roll over
letting all that concerns me fall to the side
Ananda

My body levitates upwards,
crown high like me
and OM seals my prayer
"Namaste"

All those things I thought I needed to do
worried about, was distracted by
are left in the cracks of the floor
I leave this womb refreshed

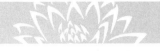

The Oak

Over the bridge,
Down stillnessway
Spring light slants, shades,
Lampfire elongated like sky-drippings
A treatise on the phenomena of the unleafed forest
Shiny-eyed wonder-canyons,
Exploding ancient gibberish bellowed on bird tongue,
Decoding winter
Chunks of bark carving crooked silhouettes
Under low gold sun
Friend tree in the slit
By the rock-gilled protruding bank
The leafing of the trees
I sit, tucked
Sweat-backed to generous girth,
Moss skin and muscular grunt
Bank's muddy edges,
Convulsive eye-battles
Between microscopic bazaar beneath toes
And the frantic leaf-parade unfolding above
Possibility
One oak,
Still gripping winter's wilted leaves
December's gloomy garments,
Convincing smile
Mute, rigid, defiant to spring's resurrection
Reminds me of the evergreens I am not
And rope swings tied to a certain solitude
Disguised as serenity
Green is a smile not tinted sepia

Not old
Not past tense
Pale, grainy
Not tattered edge memory
Retired love
Green isn't cold, clear-cut, receding
Mountain's bones
Misplaced affection
Green joins the progress of the seasons
Doesn't unravel like a fluttering banner
Beating the air
Of recollection
Green doesn't know a rough winter
Admits spring
Cups her soft-lipped lobes
Around even a dim earth
Impregnated by wind
Births spirit seeds
Rings my frozen creek edges like a song
The oak
Me
Becoming as familiar as our backward bending heart bows
Hanging onto old robes
Giving in to this convincing
Harvest of gravity
The oak
Me
Staring in the face
Diminishing sunset

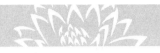

City of Seagulls

I long to be as still as the seagulls
that congregate along the surf.
Sunbathing and meditating
on the subtle breeze
sifting through their feathers.

Gazing out towards the mass
of sand with a high chin
and erect chest.
They just seem so sure of themselves.

And on two toothpick like legs
they manage to never waver or wobble
when the waves crash their way.

Hands Held High

Hands held high
Fold and bend
Strettttttch

Curve like a snake
Curl like a Child
REleaaaase

Somewhere between my triangle pose
and my downward dog I forgot about work
and lost my cares about my family and friends

Perhaps it was on the bridge that my thoughts disappeared
and reappeared with greater clarity and purpose
as I stood still as a tree.

Closed eyes dissolved the mask that I wear
to keep people and things at a distance
so I can pretend to be separate and distinct
an inner smile connected my heart beat
to the rhythm of the earth
and reverberated through each breath

Absent was the audible sound of the OM
so many erroneously correlate to a new age practice
Present was the pulse of oneness and resonance
of my heart chakra
as it opened like a flower and gave fuel to the eternal life force
that spanned beyond all of the ages
and gave rise to the collective OM
which can be only heard
if you listen from within.

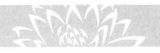

Circumvent

Think of the winter birds
that brave high cold
and northern winds,
walk for miles and miles
on end
with one egg waiting
for their icy return.
One chance
at new life.

Survival.

Think of their black and white
love dance
on times you feel pity
for your human experience.

Your broken heart.

Your triumphs and failures
that circumvent
the globe.

Think of the relativity of the words
sacrifice.
harsh.

Turn yourself into an animal
and laugh at all this chatter.

Service

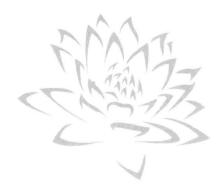

I could die here
Make my limbs a tree
Place each thought in a leaf
Fix my posture,
So my grandchildren's backs are straight.

HawaH

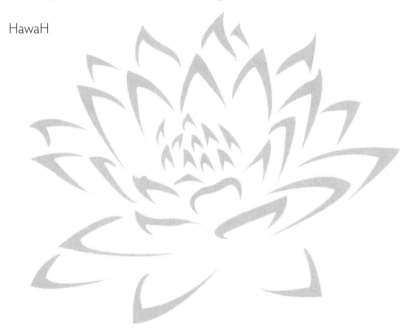

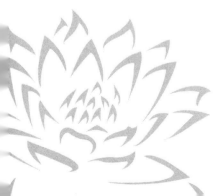

Dharma Pearls

No More Complications

If things are complicated,
be assured that you have become a stranger to your soul.
Endlessly asking how, when, who. . .
is turning away from spirit,
who quietly waits with all the answers and whimsy you need
to fully shine. Why choose complicated?
That's one more complication,
one more turning away from the simple beauty of Being.
Cast aside the complications and embrace
the quiet love that binds you to all.

Joyous

Searching outside of myself
true satisfaction remains just beyond reach.
Strange.
Returning to a vibrant inner world,
immerses me in the beauty
that I had been searching for all along.
Now that beauty is everywhere,
even in the places where I had previously seen
nothing wonderful.
Enriched by the inner light of wisdom
all longings are joyously satisfied.
Life is again an infinite celebration.
Thank Goodness.

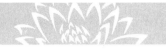

Unlock Your Locks

Mind is the key that either locks you in the prison
of your own creation
or frees you to play in Nature's exquisite
and boundless landscape.
It is easy not to see that your mind
isn't inclined toward peace.
Penetrate beyond its surface however
and access the Majestic universe,
the answers to all questions and a path through any obstacle.
Meditate to train your mind
day after day and awaken
its spectacular capacities.

Lost Socks

Stuck is a sign that you've stopped tuning
to your endlessly inventive, curious, wise
and unpredictable soul.
Don't wait to figure out why
you are not honoring your Self.
Unburden yourself of your laments,
all those lost socks you used to love,
so your life again becomes what it was meant to be:
an original, never ending song that lifts all beings.

Real Living
In meditation I tiptoe, some days soar,
into the world of the unmanifest.
Words can never fully portray this landscape of Grace,
but I can tell you that you could search endlessly
in the world of things and not have a clue about the power,
beauty and brilliance that lies beyond it.
It's hard to imagine living,
really living, without having tasted heaven.
That is why we stop to sense what everything has come from.

Ceaseless Kisses
In life's sea of hassles and troubles we search for Grace.
Most look where they can find it:
pleasure, even if it's the kind that has no staying power.
Seekers comb for it,
knowing that its rays beam brightly
during certain phases of the swinging pendulum of mind.
The sage sees Grace's ceaseless blessing everywhere.
What hardship?
Life's a Divine embrace,
like so many sweet kisses from Eternity that never stop.

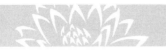

Fuel Your Spark

Things standing in your way?
Take heart.
It's part of being human.
The sages counseled,
no matter the goal—sacred or mundane—
power is key to traversing your impediments.
Tantra says lightening is already in your bottle.
Take responsibility for the gift.
The right teacher, practice, and sacrificing your distractions
will make you a lightening rod,
able to zap what stands in the way
of the treasures you seek.

Surrender

The tree has no choice
but to be tossed by the wind,
belted by hail,
scorched by the sun.
Her roots go so deep
that it doesn't matter.
The changing seasons
are no burden;
her branches yield
and her leaves fall
to nourish her another year.
And with each turn of the earth
she rises closer to the light of the sun.
And with each turn of the earth
her roots go deeper,
until at last she falls
without struggle
back into her Mother's waiting arms.

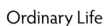

Ordinary Life

My ordinary life will sometimes tell
Me that I need to rush through dinner, or
Fill empty space with words or numb my mind
With movies, facebook, junkfood, or more wine.
And yet my ordinary life of snow,
Soup, fire, grass, sun, rabbit, cat, book, and sleep
Needs space in which to happen and be felt.
In breath, the being and the doing merge.

Like a Japanese tea ceremony,
A preparation and event itself,
All the moment needs is my attention
For each gesture to be graceful, to brew
A tea both delicate and bold, just as
Wholesome in the making as the taking.

Whole

Just as I tell myself I've arrived. . .
As I've breathed with mindful sensitivity into the placement of
My feet, legs, hips, torso, neck, head, & arms
Just as I become my pose, tasting perfection. . .

The tiniest, insistent urge to move visits.

Exploring, deeply in the center of continuous breath;
Inquiring, I inhale & lengthen, exhale & soften.
I spread the toes of one foot farther apart,
Plant the heel of the other more solidly on the earth.

Rooting through soles of feet,
Radiating from center, I engage & draw focus
Discovering one place. . .one small place
Where I can let go—

In that instant an invitation arises, I accept, &

Subtly shifting my hips. . .
I am transformed!
Space, buoyancy, & ease bloom
From this cultivated ground.

Eyes closed, air caressing skin,
Senses heighten.
Conscious of the Grace that flows
Here, in this moment

I am Whole.

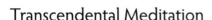

Transcendental Meditation

Sitting in a corner, cross leg down
I celebrate subconscious mind to be
On the centre of transcendental eye
I mutter a holy mantra
To bring my roaming attention
which tries to slip away
like fish from the grip of hand
to reemerge into the pond
filled and flowing with water of illusion.

I let loose all my limbs
As if they were not mine
And I contemplate upon
self composed darkness outside
only one dwelling inside to illumine.

Awakened

Nothing works.
The usual things

that acted so well
on other days

are left alone.
What kind of truth

tries to establish
itself through you?

The voice of the past
is heard and responded to.

A voice deep
in recollections,

self-deceits. You
never know how

you would act
tomorrow, now that

the past has
taken hold

of miracles, cryptic
histories of the self.

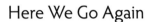

Here We Go Again

an investigation took place
        on my cushion this morning
a dozen suspect thoughts in a lineup
the witness identified every one

exposed, they fell silent
though guilty of impersonation
        they were harmless and released

then the whole place faded
as a convincing dream dissolves
it disappeared—a curl of smoke in the wind
and a shimmering sea of pictureless sound
        emerged in its place

am i forever bound by these phantoms—
shadowy figures whispering clever lies from alleyways

let me press my head even closer to the floor
take refuge in the secret hand
        that somehow threads a needle in this darkness
that creates a path for me
        even when i run in the wrong direction

let that boundless heart be my last home

God's Waiting Room

There can be no appointment with God
None that we can arrange
The best we can do is take shelter
In His waiting room
Knowing if we stay long enough
He's bound to pass through

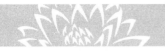

Jeremy Frindel

You

there is no other

208

Bird

Our wings get broken
our feathers, mangled and plucked
but we can still Fly. . .

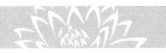

Un Poema Por Un Amor Desconocido

La vida es una pesadilla hermosa.

Hay felicidad y tristeza, sonrisas y lagrimas,
ganancias y perdidas.

Pero cuando tu me tocas, lo olvido todo,
y el alma respira otra vez.

A Poem For An Unknown Love

Life is a beautiful nightmare.

There is happiness and sadness, smiles and tears,
gains and losses.

But when you touch me, I forget it all,
and my soul breathes
once again.

Niralambaya Tejase

Pining for the relative existence
a process with no abbreviations. . .
no alterations, leaving me with sleeves short and a split sense
of misguided adorations. . .
who does assume this form of reality. . .
consciousness and bliss
while the world around us is absent and not at peace. . .
hard to keep my posture from my pose
while my understanding is laced with omnipresent suffering. . .
seduced by the conceptual practice of healing
when we advertise the plight of mankind
every hour on the hour. . .
intermittent commercials
selling me ease and solutions to problems
that have been illuminated
in vein by the truth at hand. . .
we are where we stand. . .
just as much as where we sit and what we sit with. . .
and the process. . .
the process to a true understanding of freedom
that requires no others to fall. . .
the cosmic imbalance that teaches us to surrender. . .
in a culture that has taught us that surrendering is a process
of elimination not a process of salvation. . .
sacrifice and devotion. . .

Pulling Strings

Love lines falling from the sky
Pinned to limbs, heart and voice
direct me please
so I may speak act and play
with unfettered compassion and grace.

Look Inside

If I only look inside, I see nothing
If I observe inside, I find the universe

If I find nothing, I find everything
If I don't love anyone, I truly love everyone

If I sit and listen in my universe
listening I give you my compassion
Don't ask my advice, I place it
in your path, don't ask my judgement
I only observe

If you find a friend in me
I am on the right path
because I have attracted you

If I love you, but don't need you, be sure
my love is sincere
If you love me, but can live without me, I am sure
you really love me

Although we are two rivers living separately from one another,

One day we will both end up in the same ocean.

Into Me

Racing pulse as the sweat drips down
My petrified bones unmovable
Like a sculpture it screams let me go
Out of this space I find my eyes
Open to a black curtain tickling
Painfully teasing me are its ties
To my head that go left to right
Touching nothing but feeling everything
That is there and not there
But is here and getting near
To take me away forever theirs
A rock under my hand, smooth
The surface is, hurting and soothing
My fear is reaching its peak
Into my heart the drumming
Sounds deafening, healing, beautiful
Lightness lifts me up, loosening
The stiffness, no more
Lying to myself, it's pointless
To resist the beauty of flight
At this hour soaring high
Are the clouds beneath me
Is the body and the home
I thought was mine but I now see
Up here and down there
It's not me because I'm everywhere
I see it's me, and it's you too
That I see when I took the journey
Into me, suddenly
I understood.

Bound

We tie ourselves up in thoughts and beliefs
So tight that our convictions clench down
a solid structure of gospel
Never to be unwound

Or we might have to question
The binder twine that holds us together
In solid form

So easily cut loose
That if free
Our inner parts would breathe into a wildness
so pure it must be god

So we dance
Between bondage and freedom
Not certain which one is better

Hoping that each time we unwind
It won't be our undoing
But an opening to something better

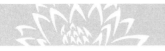
The Simplicity of Breath

It is enough now, the blue blue sea
And the whites of her eyes and cloud
Like sheets of glass on high.

I will take you there, where you have been,
And already are, the place
Not of worship or want, or knowing
But the simplicity of breath
And your light chest heaving
Like swells of the sea
And the taste of spray on your tongue.

Giant Earplugs

The mountains this morning
Are giant earplugs
Deafening all sound
In the canyon of my mind.
The sky is thin
But a sheet of glass
Reflecting back to me
The pitter-patter of my thoughts.
Ozone.

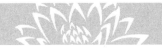

It

The sort of it is It.
The it of it is It.
The all of it is It.

I'm Lucky

I'm lucky to be of the Iroquois
Who have, they say, twelve souls that they enjoy.
I have a pagan soul that I employ
About the skies adorned with hope I scan.
I have a Christian soul, a Jewish plan,
A Muslim soul and one Samaritan.
My Hindu soul clashes not with the Jain,
My Buddhist with my Taoist soul in vain.
Confucianist is the last soul I name,
Besides the Druid that I love to claim.
The twelfth soul is the first, a secret song
Outside the lays of righteousness and wrong
Of the great world traditions: it's my soul
That's hidden in You, my Beloved and goal.

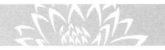

Revelation

It's not about them or us, or even about you;
it is about me, about
taking of myself
setting boundaries
connecting while remaining independent
It is about accepting responsibility
for my own insecurities.

Sadhana Reveals

a curious introduction and a bunch of awkward firsts
gave way to a shape, a space, a movement, a rhythm
re-learning my breath, re-learning my body, realizing myself

comfort in this familiar ritual of breath and body
this grand ancient mala of pearls, worn yet casts light
enlivened in the sharing, made new in the practice

this journey with a path endlessly inward, constantly deeper
beckons with fiercely eager
yearning
yet profoundly tranquil calm
rewrites my life, unfolding as moments of sparkling truth

both private and fully revealed
in this reunion with my beloved divine
i see my true self within the sacred sound

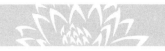

Home

I sit in Lotus
and wonder
as I did that day dreaming
in Ojito with a white hawk on shoulder
what home meant
where it was
and I disappeared
blending into oneness of wind, sage, pine
sandstone, sun, and ancient sea
home again
in the heart of this life.

Star. . .

As I swim to the bare unconscious
naked and pure
my five star talisman within
I am reaching with my own hand
my own will
within reach nearing my fingertips
with magnetic tides pulling us together
with the five directions
and the sun's reflections
my dreams are attainable
the unconscious coming to the surface
a reflection of the inner and outer
a masculine and feminine encounter. . .

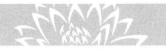

Flying at Night

From up here, I can see clearly.

Faint flickering lights hint at the path of a winding road
That stretches out across the land.
Dice thrown on the table of the night.

The light of a town glares in the distance,
A burning ember held in the black palm of the night.
People are drawn to this cold fire
to live near others of their kind.

I can see their lives from here.

Another faint spark flickers
in the dark distance.
An outpost at the edge of what men know. . .

Let me live there,
on that edge that swallows men
and their electricity.
Embracing all in silent wonder.

Fearless.

Gigantic.

Invisible.

When They Ask About Your Gods

when they ask you about your gods,

tell them you believe in the white blaze
of a star, burst from its bud
in the clear sky of a frozen night.

tell them about the silent whispers that rise
from the deep black waters of your soul
and flow through any ordinary moment.

and tell them how there are no ordinary moments.

how life in every second is moving wildly
over this canvas, across this landscape, to an unknown sea.

then tell them about your mother's voice:
how it cracked exquisitely that time she
touched her heart and spoke your name.

how she never taught you to abandon your seeking,
but to fall always and everywhere
towards the center of your being.

when they ask you, tell them these things.
tell them how god reaches out for god.

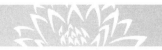

Searching

it's easy
to catch me
in the act
of
searching.
my key
my words
my soul.
i am a harbinger of
drawers
left open.
and i wonder at things
like:
what keeps a bird
up
what keeps a heart
down
why the sea returns to shore
each time
it is rejected.
at the quiet lift
of early morning, why,
in the orange light
of rising
i've
been known to forget
the forms
of name and place
as thoughts rise up like springtime mountains—
carry me over treetops
through forests
and out to the open sea.
only to find the thing
i've been searching for
has also been searching
for me.

At Your Service
(*Translated from Spanish by Catherine Prescott and HawaH*)

In the name of yesterday, today and tomorrow,
I ask my great strength awakened,
to protect, care, teach, and serve,
and from this day forth
To stand with you in the face of injustice

Warrior ancestor return

How long is the way
till the hand of courage
Knocks on my door
I need not walk this path alone

When I open

Worlds, lives, years, reincarnations
clear our path, dissolve our actions
to understand life's lessons

Strength, power, fame, fortune and beauty
are worldly things longed for. . .
When forgetting true happiness and success
are beyond the material world

Protect, care, teach, and serve,
a way of life,
to share my love and feel one
with all my brothers and sisters, until my last heartbeat.
Begins again.

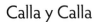

Calla y Calla

I am a scale by which your body floats lithe and buoyant under
the dense canopy of mossy live oak shading the Amphitheater
Shouldn't we perform our defiance for onlookers
jogging between rest stops
fixing our positions into stone?

How remarkable you stretch above me
Gravity is a state of mind, beyond thought,
anchored in a belief
that centers of mass flex then break
when stressed beyond vision

I have fallen asleep to your voice,
but you misread
my conduct as dismissive.
Your voice is sanctuary,
a place I can inhabit,
a warm shroud.
Now I am about to fall into
the emptiness of your possibility,
folded into your arms,
bending the air, instructing
my body to lift the air with you,
like the meniscus, an insoluble needle,
retracing the sonograph
of our diminished selves,
a crepuscular horizon, we are transparent

Where else can we meet in winter,
and orbit a persuasive constellation,
listening to the quietude of its clusters,
and maybe ease the ampolleta passing
judgment over our time together.

Effluence

And she unfolded.
Just like a letter.
Reaching and flipping and turning,
until she lay flat on her back.
Chest open.
Palms up.
Her words for the world to see.
Creases and tears across her cheeks.
Scars and smudges across her skin.
Misspelled poetry in private places;

curse words and professions exposed.
Her heart beat open upon her ribcage,

revealing her depth of life
in painted colors.
Its value bubbling over in streams of brilliant hues.
Washing away the tepid floor boards
that hold her down.
Releasing a resplendent light

of self protection.

So strong and calm,
that her reflection
matched that of the sunshine
that illuminated downwards.

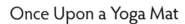

Once Upon a Yoga Mat

Once upon a yoga mat
With myself I simply sat
I put my ass upon the floor
I found my breath and connected my core
Inhale
Exhale
Forward bend
Deep inside things start to mend
Finding space between my toes
breathing in through my nose
Stacking my bones
Strong and still
I start to exert free will
A simple choice
That's mine to make
Simply shine bright
Real not fake
How I am feeling
What I express
Things I uncover
Drenched and a mess

The Ranting and Raving Old Monk

The ranting and raving old beloved monk,
covered with flowing butterscotch robes—

What if the expanding universe had shrunk,
into scientific matters he probes—

And the troubles of this world he contemplates,
the devastation driven all by greed—

No light possible if everyone hates,
attachment to the self, a bitterweed—

Clearly though, it's always been the same,
he says, even the rarest sparkling stars—

The Gandhis and Kings couldn't fan the flame,
remove the affliction, or iron the scars—

Racing in vain to unscramble life's clues,
for simply looking inside, most refuse.

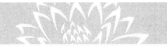

Love Poem for Shakti

the heart is a place
of mystery
green
and fragrant,
wild with vines
and tears,
oceans and

starsalan
an empty hallway
of drums
a horizon of sunsets,
swingsets
echoing with
the unstruck sound
the heart
is a chamber
of bells

i open it like a drawer
for you
like a temple door
carved in wood
covered in thumbprints
weighing ten thousand pounds
yet it grows light as breath
for you
breeze
swings open with a sigh
silent as prayer

and you boldly enter
with your highbeams
and your tigerskin on
a whole marching band
parade with floats
follows you in

it's a full-on celebration here
in the field
of the heart

when you enter

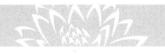

Skinned Knee

ask and you shall receive
but be careful what you wish for

i wanted liberation in london
they lost my luggage
i found myself alone
surrounded by yankees and brits

i wanted ananda in canada
to camp at an ashram
too much chanting
esoteric philosophies
and a mean swami later
i was back home in bed, depressed

i wanted californian change
found out, yes, there is such a thing
as too much yoga
and there are both zen centers and christian radicals
in the city by the bay

i wanted to soak up mexico
to eat sandia with frida
came home with a souvenir
en mi corazon
and one in my intestines

i wanted india in my skin
fell to my knees and scraped the left one
the dhamma nazis threw saffron-colored powder on my little
wound
it didn't hurt
but i cried quiet tears that had been waiting years to reach
the surface

this moment is perfect
every one is
equanimity tattooed inside my forehead
gratitude for spiders and saffron and dhamma

what will you ask for?
what will you receive?

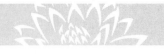

Dark and Light

dark and light are next door neighbors
dark is the desert with scrub brush and rattlesnakes
light is she who wears a satin gown that glows
she floats on a translucent veil of fluttering doves
her feet never leave the ground
the elements move through her like dancing waves
sometimes tidal ones
and she stays completely still
dark is fear
sticky
sweaty
light is beauty
brilliance
love
a warm radiating sunshine
it encompasses with nourishment
dark encompasses
with a windowless stuffy arrogance
a dim future
short sighted vision
stuffed pockets of stolen dreams
both live inside of me
they are the fertile ground of consciousness
each day I go to them
and I ask if we can all work together
can we meet in the middle
right in the center
beyond "my house or yours"
where the door between is wide open
and the magical mystery is queen

she passes through
back and forth
with the grace of blue heron
eating brunch over there and tea over here
she becomes an honored guest, no longer in prison
she feeds me words that tumble out like jewels
the most precious kind
like ripe pomegranate seeds
sweet and delicious
leaving little stains of ruby
on my shirt
when dark and light get along,
I float down the river
on a boat fit for a queen
and I rest in the outrageous delight
of the unfolding heart.

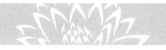

Kali Ma

In the bushes I lay there dead
exploded
like shimmering stardust
melted wax
a sailor's knot
your face right up close
familiar
with eyes wide open
a mouth full of space
and a garland of letters around your waist
the bright sun brings it to light
In the center
the midline between
who I was and
will be
I sat there with the seed in my heart
that never changed
even as my limbs were strewn
amidst the heap of days gone by
you sat there right in front
cheering me on
as I crumbled to
pieces of whole
and cried tears
of infinite sadness
infinite joy
and everything else
in between.

Sunset Sandhya

Solstice Canyon is the edge
that has dissolved all my practices.

Sitting here at sunset,
the peak of the day where breath hovers,

a presence permeates this valley

ancestors
vivid colors,
the scent of wild sage, fennel, rosemary,
the brillant fireball of the Sun
the ocean becoming sky on the horizon
a hawk soaring without effort
making One song of this moment.

As the sky melts into orange, purple and blue,
my eyes bathe in sublime beauty
my practices wash down my cheeks

no-thing is left
only the breath dancing
in everything.

Acknowledgements

My deepest gratitude to our ancestors, upon your shoulders we stand, and may you continue to use me as a vessel for your spirit and passion, strength and wisdom, beauty and grace. This book is your reflection and now our shared dreams.

This project is bigger than just one person, and honestly, it's bigger than just a book. There were so many people involved in helping bring it to fruition. *The Poetry of Yoga* started as a workshop series until my dear friend Katie Capano planted the seed in my brain to turn it into a book. Over the two years, from idea to manifestation, she was always my first opinion. From there it was a snowball of amazing volunteers, supporters, and kindred spirits helping to make it a reality.

Indispensable through the whole process was Laura Berol. In the beginning of 2011, she came on as a One Common Unity fellow, assigned to this fundraising initiative. She helped manage and direct communications for the project, organized databases, and created outreach trackers. She was the only one, other than me, who read all the submissions that came in through our website. Most importantly, she was so unbelievably gracious with her time and heart.

Also, great thanks to Bethany Wichman and Chivonnie Gius-Meekins, for their support in the office and belief in my dream that this book would raise money for One Common Unity youth programs! Interns Ariel Saidman and Albatoul Basha were instrumental during the infant stages of this project.

In the final phase, Max C. Gilbert was tremendous and meticulous in completing the layout and design for Volume 1. Bill Tipper pushed in the clutch when he offered one of his gorgeous photographs for the front cover in the last moments before production. His work is divine (www.billtipper.com).

A special thank you to Sarah of Massey Media who spent a year helping me sculpt a story arc and National Tour for the workshop series back in 2010. Jill Kianka of Vico Rock Media provided amazing web development and design of *The Poetry of Yoga* site.

The wonderful Erin Weston worked diligently to record and produce audio and video. And her colleague Michael Lindley assisted her in putting together the informational video announcing the book launch.

As I burned the midnight oil, there were numerous people who stepped up by helping with suggestions, edits, revisions, recording audio, producing media broadcasts, and PR, including: Sia Tiambi Barnes, Doug Swenson, Radhakrishna Kasat, Chelsea Edgett, Mikuak Rai, Sharon Gannon, Sianna Sherman, Ellie Walton, Jessica Durivage, Diane Ferraro, Rod Stryker, Joanne Jagoda, Bob Weisenberg, Shiva Rea, Debra & Ian Mishalove, Lalita Noronha-Blob, Utamu Onaje, Luke Shors, and Madhuri Kasat.

Then finally, I met Steve Scholl, publisher of White Cloud Press. He saw great potential in all I was doing and was so moved by the project that he offered to publish it under the White Cloud name. Both him and Christy Collins, production manager of White Cloud Press, were fantastic in creating a new layout and design for this new edition of Volume 1 and taking it out to the masses!

Infinite love to my parents and family who have always been supportive of all my crazy ideas; and, of course, to all of you! The hundreds upon hundreds of people who sent in poetry, shared the word with their friends, and lent their voices to this massive project.

About the Editor

HawaH has dedicated his life to teaching about solutions to violence and ways to peace, and has traveled to over 35 countries to facilitate interactive workshops, dialogues, perform poetry, teach yoga, and speak with those interested in creating a caring, sustainable, and equitable world. He has worked as an Americorps big brother in one of Washington, D.C.'s most under-resourced neighborhoods, and also as an R.F.K. Memorial Foundation fellow as a special representative to the United Nations and the World Conference Against Racism.

HawaH is co-founder and executive director of One Common Unity, a non-profit organization that inspires non-violent culture through education, music and media. For 3 years he directed the Peaceable Schools Program in D.C.'s largest public high school—specifically developing leadership skills of youth and assisting them in dealing with trauma through Alternatives to Violence, Deep Breathing & Yoga classes.

Over the years, HawaH has trained thousands of teachers in the principles of social-emotional learning and has regularly featured as a speaker, performer and workshop presenter for People to People International, the Congressional Youth Leadership Council and the Children's Defense Fund's Freedom Schools. A spoken word poet known as *Everlutionary* and an artist of a diverse collection of paintings and photographs, he has authored four books, produced three documentary films, and released two musical CD's.

Other works by HawaH

Books
Trails: Trust Before Suspicion (non-fiction travel novel) — 2001

Escape Extinction (essays and poetry) — 2003

zerONEss (poetry and prose) — 2005

Documentary Films
A Weigh With Words — 2007

The MLK Streets Project — 2011

Fly By Light — 2015

CDs:
Survival for All Of Us — 2008

CALL — 2010

Online
www.EVERLUTIONARY.net — 2000

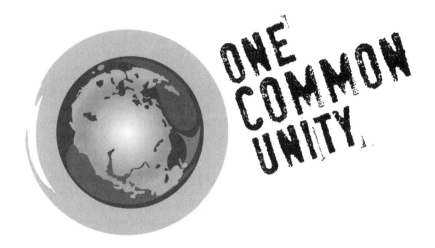

One Common Unity is a grassroots 501(c)3 non-profit organization. Since the year 2000, they have been supporting and inspiring a movement for peace education and the building of a nonviolent culture through music, media and art.

For more information about their pioneering initiatives please visit www.OneCommonUnity.org

50% of proceeds from this book are donated to their work.

www.ThePoetryOfYoga.com

www.Facebook.com/ThePoetryOfYoga

Questions, feedback, collaborations, or suggestions?
Email us at poetryofyoga@gmail.com